NEW HAVEN PUBLIC LIBRARY

3 5000 09433 1203

W9-CNI-937

ALSO BY SUE FLEMING

Buff Brides

Buff Moms-to-Be

Buff Moms

FASHIONABLY
BUFF

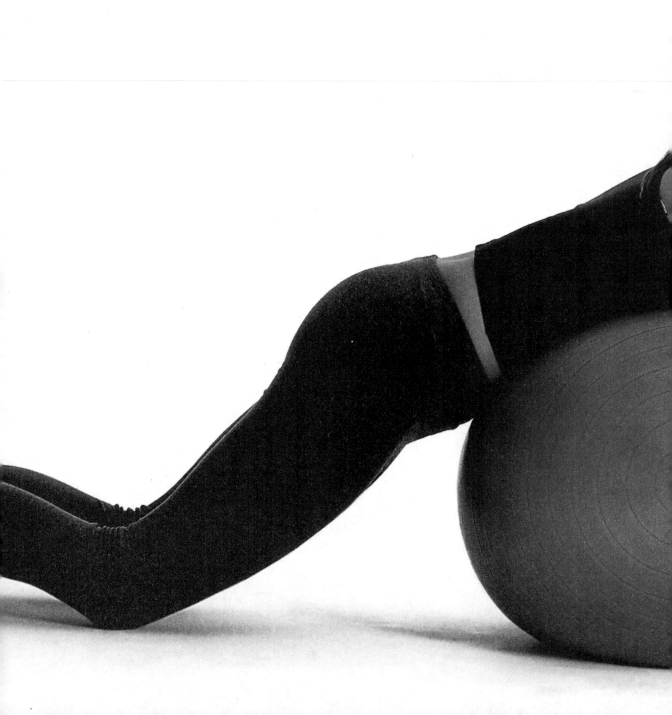

FASHIONABLY BUFF

SUE FLEMING

Essential Workouts for Looking

Great in Anything You Wear

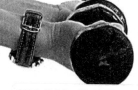

VILLARD BOOKS NEW YORK

613.704 FLEMING
Fashionably buff
 :essential workouts fo
35000094331203
MITCHELL

Author's Note: This book proposes a program of exercise recommendations for the reader to follow. However, you should consult a qualified medical professional (and, if you are pregnant, your ob-gyn) before starting this or any other fitness program. As with any diet or exercise program, if at any time you experience any discomfort, stop immediately and consult your physician.

A Villard Books Trade Paperback Original

Copyright © 2007 by Buff, Inc.

Photographs copyright © 2007 by Kelly Campbell

All rights reserved.

Published in the United States by Villard Books,
an imprint of The Random House Publishing Group,
a division of Random House, Inc., New York.

VILLARD and "V" CIRCLED Design are registered
trademarks of Random House, Inc.

ISBN 978-0-8129-7225-2

Library of Congress Cataloging-in-Publication data
is available.

Printed in the United States of America

www.villard.com

9 8 7 6 5 4 3 2 1

Book design by Jo Anne Metsch

To my friends and family

CONTENTS

INTRODUCTION

S o spring has arrived. You open up your closet and are over-
come with dread. Next to the cashmere sweaters and wool
pants is the sectioned-off corner that hasn't been touched in months,
or even years; clothing casualties of spring and summer are roped off
like a crime scene. Bright sleeveless blouses and tank tops along with
sexy summer dresses mock you with body-exposing styles. Then your
eyes come to rest on that stack of blue jeans that sits in the corner col-
lecting dust, taunting you, waiting for you to shed those inches so you
can get them back on again. You've been meaning all winter to work on
getting the perfect butt to fit your favorite, neglected pair. Yeah. Right.

If you're like most women, your first thought is probably *Ugh—I
have to go to the gym.* And your second thought is probably *I can't.* The
fact is, most people don't have the time to go to the gym and would
rather learn a brief, intense exercise routine they can do at home.

My clients have taught me that there is nothing more intimidating
than a closet full of (scary) too-small clothes—and, of course, no confidence to wear them. But *Fashionably Buff* is the answer to these
problems. This helpful, fun guide targets all the essential areas of your
body to ensure that you look hot and fit in everything from your favorite jeans to your little black dress. Spot workouts specially de-

signed to be easy and manageable will shape you up so you can tear that DO NOT CROSS yellow police tape out of your closet!

In the pages ahead, you're going to learn how to turn your home into a personal gym to help you achieve your fitness goals. You're going to learn specific exercises that will help you tone and trim those areas of your body to help you look buff for the essential wardrobe. You're going to learn specific motivating techniques to help you achieve an awesome body, better health, and increased confidence—all while having some fun!

Exercise does not have to be complicated to be effective. But it does take commitment. I've noted throughout my years as a fitness instructor that everyone does best by setting small, attainable goals. And although results do not come overnight, improvement is pretty much a sure thing if you follow my exercises. I'll help you make reasonable goals and achieve them; then you'll never be afraid of a tank top again! But goals require the right exercises, and that's where this book comes in—it will be your buff bible!

The series of workouts should take you only fifteen to twenty minutes. Feel free to combine workouts for an even longer session. The keys are to do the exercises with correct form and to do each routine four times per week.

You will also notice that many of the exercises stimulate multiple muscle groups. I'm all about multitasking and getting the most from your valuable time. Most people waste precious minutes during their workouts. This book will teach you how to maximize your time with efficient and successful planning.

FASHIONABLY
BUFF

PART I

Dos and Don'ts for Choosing Clothes

CHAPTER 1

LOOKING GOOD ON TOP

BODY TYPES: WORKING WITH WHAT YOU'VE GOT!

Despite countless apparel choices, female consumers remain frustrated in their search for the perfect-fitting outfit. The shape of a female body is referred to as a *figure,* and the shape of a male body is frequently referred to as a *physique.* I think the word *figure* just puts more pressure on women because it implies that we must conform to society's view of the ideal "figure"—something created, imagined, and sculpted.

The fact is, we are all different. Some people have brown hair and others are blond; some folks are tall and slim, while others are short and stocky. And some women are curvy, while others are angular. So how in the world can we expect the same clothes off the rack to fit us all the same way? It's obviously impossible.

When was the last time you had your measurements taken so that a garment fit you perfectly? For some of you, it was most likely when you were fitted for a bridal gown. For most of you, I'll bet—never! Being fussed over in multiple bridal fittings bears no resemblance to most women's everyday clothes-shopping experience, but many women do wish that the clothes they bought fit their bodies well. Unfortunately, this is rare. But there *are* tricks for choosing the most flattering cut for your body shape. So once you determine what sort of body you have, you're one step closer to looking fashionably buff!

The area where body fat is predominantly stored essentially determines body shape. There are primarily two types of body shapes: the pear shape and the apple shape. I will describe what is meant by *pear-shaped* and *apple-shaped* and how to dress to flatter each of these body types.

To see whether you are pear-shaped, obtain your waist–hip ratio (also known as trunk fatness). Divide your waist measurement by your hip measurement. If the ratio is 0.8 inch or less, then you are pear-shaped. If the ratio is more than 0.8 inch, then you are apple-shaped.

Pears, or endomorphs, are generally women who store fat below the waistline on their hips, thighs, and bottoms, as opposed to their stomachs and midsections. Such fat being stored on the thighs often leads to cellulite, or those thin trails of white lines on the skin also called stretch marks. The upper torso is relatively slim in comparison with the lower parts of the body, with shoulders and bust being narrow compared with the hips. Pear-shaped women are commonly viewed as bottom-heavy, with well-defined waists.

Apples are women who have wide torsos (full bust, waist, and upper back), as they store body fat around the midsection (stomach, abdomen, and chest). Such women have relatively slim thighs and upper legs. Apple-shaped women often have a top-heavy appearance, with a bust and midriff bigger than their hips, a prominent tummy, and a flat bottom.

Ultimately, you cannot change your fundamental body shape. Your basic body type is greatly outside your control—more to do with DNA and your childhood lifestyle than anything else. So if you are over eighteen and reading this, you are what you are, although you can fine-tune what you already have.

Research is ongoing as to what causes women to fall into either category. However, apples do tend to find it easier to shed excess body weight than pears, as fatty deposits around the stomach area will break down far more quickly than fat stored on the hips and thighs. Thus with a sensible diet and exercise regime, the increased health risks for an apple can be counteracted, and an apple-shaped woman can change her overall shape. Pears will lose weight from their upper body more easily than from their hips and thighs and will always maintain their same basic pear shape.

Each of us has a unique figure, and we can enhance our appearance by drawing attention to our best features. Here are some simple dos and don'ts when choosing your next outfit.

WHAT TO WEAR ON TOP FOR THE PEAR SHAPE

If you're bottom-heavy or pear-shaped, avoid too-baggy tops or too-tight tops. Baggy tops will make you look large and sloppy; tight tops will make you look out of proportion to your hips. Fitted T-shirts and tanks work well, and V-necks draw attention to your face. Jackets and blazers should hit at the widest point of your hips. Depending on your height, that point could fall anywhere from right below the waist to midthigh.

When choosing a dress, look for something that cinches in at the waist and flares out slightly over the hips and thighs. Sleeveless and

NOT ENOUGH ON TOP?

If you'd like to look heavier on the top, bulky and bouffant styles will add some definition to a slight frame. Curved, horizontal, and diagonal lines will also help.

strapless dresses will look great after your Buff in a Tank Top workout (see page 75). An empire- or raised-waist dress brings the eye up away from your lower body.

WHAT TO WEAR ON TOP FOR THE APPLE SHAPE

The apple-shaped body is usually softer around the middle and has heavier breasts, narrower hips, and slimmer legs. Again, you want to keep people's eyes off the problem areas—this is a great time to show off your legs and cleavage! Women with large breasts must decide how they want to emphasize (or not) their chests.

Choosing a Smart Top for the Apple Shape

When picking out the right outfit, stay away from supertight tops, which emphasize larger breasts. On the flip side, wearing baggy blouses only makes you look heavier. Look for fabrics that offer a little stretch. V-necks, boat necks, and turtlenecks are the most flattering. Show off your nice arms with a sleeveless shirt or tank top; compliment your large breasts with a structured strapless top. And try not to wear anything that has puffy sleeves!

NECKLINES FOR YOUR FACE AND BODY TYPE

You know the basics: The right necklines flatter your shoulders and bust. But did you know that a cleverly chosen neckline can balance out your face shape, too? Necklines are a critical styling component in your wardrobe because they can flatter (or worsen) your face shape and upper body. Necklines can make or break a style. Here are some pointers for selecting necklines that suit you.

STOCK UP YOUR STYLE

After you've determined the necklines that look good on you, stock up on them when they're in fashion. The less common necklines, such as cowl necks and boat necks, tend to cycle in and out of style, so get your hands on them when they're abundant and you'll have more designs to choose from.

Necklines for Your Face Shape

When choosing the necklines that flatter your face shape, you're trying to find a delicate balance. The rule is to select necklines that are "opposite" your face shape. For example, if you have a round, full face, you'll want to elongate it with deep and plunging necklines. V-necks and V-shaped scoop necks are perfect for this job. A long face needs widening, so is complimented by off-the-shoulder styles and tube tops. Square, angular jaws need to be softened by a lacy or scoop neckline, while women with small, elfish chins do best in boat necks or wide scoop necks.

- **Round-shaped faces.** Go for cowl necks, square necks, and mock turtlenecks.
- **Heart-shaped faces.** You'll want boat necks and jewel necks.
- **Long-shaped faces.** Get turtlenecks and jewel necks.
- **Oval-shaped faces.** You'll look great in almost anything!

Necklines for Your Neck and Shoulders

If you have a short or thick neck, elongate it with cowl necks, scoop necks, or V-necks. If you have a double chin, conceal it with a turtleneck.

If you're broad-shouldered, try plunging necklines such as scoop necks and V-necks, which will draw attention away from the shoulders. Avoid tight crew necks and some square necks.

Narrow-shouldered girls can wear pretty much anything. To create the illusion of broader shoulders, consider off-the-shoulder tops or halter tops with high necklines.

Necklines for Your Bust and Chest

The basic rule of thumb: The lower the neckline, the sexier it may appear—but lower necklines also tend to deemphasize bust size. So weigh the pros and cons from there.

If you are busty, opt for open-collared shirts and V-necks to minimize your chest. You can also wear off-the-shoulder styles and square necks. Avoid tight crew necks and turtlenecks.

The small-chested should go for boat necks, cowl necks, and jewel necks to add width to the upper torso.

Universal Necklines

There are some friendly necklines, styles that work on all body shapes. If you're still not sure what suits you best, go for these safe bets:

- Halter
- Scoop neck
- High neck
- Off the shoulders
- V-neck
- Round neck

CHAPTER 2

FINDING THE RIGHT BOTTOM

t's difficult to come across women who *don't* want to hide some part of their lower bodies. If you're one of the many who wants to camouflage her lower parts, choosing the right clothes will help hide problem thighs or an all-too-round bum, and help build your confidence on your way to working out.

FOR PEAR SHAPES

If you're bottom-heavy or pear-shaped, your hips are generally wider than your shoulders, and your thighs are round. When picking out something to wear, remember to accentuate the positive: a shapely waist, delicate upper body, and attractive shoulders and arms. Try to avoid skintight clothes on the bottom. A-line skirts that hit around the knee are ideal because they draw attention away from the problem areas. Miniskirts are generally a bad idea because they accentuate heavy thighs. Long skirts can make you look taller and hide thick legs.

Pant waists should fall below your natural waistline for a better fit. A straight or slightly boot-cut leg is the most flattering. You will also want to avoid patterned or light-colored pants. Cargo pants or anything that accentuates the hips are a no-no. Shorts are generally tricky, so try to stick with loose-fitting shorts or those that feature a side stripe—it will give the illusion of sleekness.

FOR APPLE SHAPES

I have four words: *Stay away from pleats!* Always choose flat, fitted pants with a lower rise. Jeans with back pockets work well, as the pockets can help define your butt—good for an apple figure. Tight jeans and pants don't work, because they only accentuate your top. This is a good time to break out the skirts that fall right above the knee.

If you're choosing a dress, remember that a one-piece may not be your best choice. Take a look at sleeveless or strapless dresses. If you're wearing a straight skirt with boots, show off a bit of leg. It will make you look less stumpy!

THE LUCKY ONES

For ectomorphs—those who are lean and narrow—wide-legged jeans, low-rise cuts, and boot cuts work best. Patch pockets and cargo pants can help fill out the hips. Anything that has curved or horizontal lines will be flattering on a slim lower body. You will look great in pencil skirts, as these tend to make you look curvier. A-lines are also great— they create curves on a straight frame. The A-line hides and highlights as needed.

CHAPTER 3

A BRIEF TANK-TOP PRIMER

D efinition of *tank top:* a short, sleeveless top with wide armholes.

Sure, sounds harmless, doesn't it? Tanks are everywhere and come in all styles; ribbed, sleek, string, athletic, sexy. But one thing is for sure: Everyone wants to expose jacked arms, not cover them up under a shirt! We know how tank tops should be worn. Not only does a toned and defined upper body look great in a tank top, but a sculpted upper body can create the illusion of a smaller and trimmed waist as well.

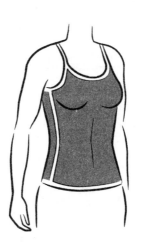

CHAPTER 4

LOOKING GOOD IN JEANS

What's all the fuss about? Gosh, it's only a butt! Well, with today's low-rise jeans showing major tummy and butt cleavage, the perfect bum is a must. And finding the perfect jeans can be a shopping nightmare. Having a couple of pairs of perfect "butt" jeans is not a luxury but a necessity. It's no secret that most of us rely on our jeans to get through the day. Many of us are as attached to our jeans as we are to our loved ones, and why not? We can dress 'em up, dress 'em down, bring 'em to work, bring 'em on a date, stroll with 'em on the weekend, cry our hearts out in 'em, test out the new heels with 'em, or pair 'em with some hot sneaks. There's nothing we can't do in our jeans, and who doesn't want to look her best in something she spends more time with than her significant other?

A SIMPLE GUIDE TO DENIM

The Rise

Rise refers to the distance from the crotch to the waistline. Some rises, of course, are lower than others. Picking the one for you may depend on your belly, your butt, and your comfort level!

Superlow

Best if you have superflat abs that you want to show off, superlow jeans also look best on petites because of the short zipper.

Low

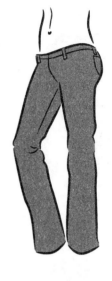

Low-rise jeans sit on your hips approximately three inches below the belly button. This is one of the styles that can look great on most body shapes.

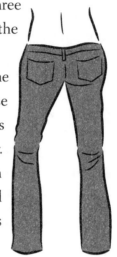

Of all the rises, this is the easiest to wear and the most comfortable. The low rise also works for those with a bigger behind. That's because the waist hits low in the back, making your butt appear smaller. Just remember that low-rise jeans tend to thicken and lengthen the waist, narrow the hips, and shorten the legs. If these are exactly the features you're trying to hide, avoid the low rise.

Classic

The classic rise is making a comeback, because it helps to hide the belly. The longer zipper looks best on taller women.

The Cut

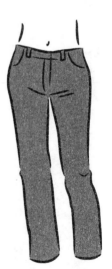

The cut and hem of your jeans make the most of your height and the length of your legs.

Cropped

Cropped jeans end somewhere between the knee and the ankle, depending on the style.

These look great on average to tall women, but not as good if you're

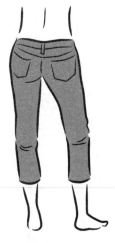

short. Wearing them can make you look much shorter than you really are. Cropped styles (pedal pushers, Capris, clam diggers) shorten your silhouette by making your hips look larger, your legs shorter, and your ankles thicker, so it's best to skip them if you're on the short and chunky side. If you are petite, you can re-hem your cropped jeans to hit in the middle of your calf so your legs look longer.

Cropped jeans look great with flip-flops, heels, or boots.

A final note: Avoid light-colored cropped jeans with cuffed bottoms, unless you are superskinny!

Straight Cut

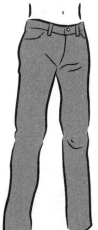

Straight-legged trouser styles can come in wide-legged cuts and slim-fitting cuts. They're great for women who have slim hips and boyish figures. Straight legs also help women with thin, long legs and a bit of a belly, because they draw attention downward. High-heeled boots and stilettos are great, as they make the legs look even longer.

If you're short or have short legs, do go ahead with slim-fitting straight-cut jeans with a higher waist to create the illusion of longer legs. Hems that end just below the ankles will elongate your legs even more. And sass up with stilettos! Shorter women should avoid wide-legged cuts. If you're blessed with height, no worries—you'll look good in either cut. Try the low-waisted kind for a sexier silhouette.

Skinny

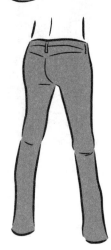

This cut is fitted all the way down to the ankles. Perfect for those with boyish frames, because the slender cut at the calves adds curves to the hips and behind, skinny jeans are also ideal for shorter females because the long leg line adds height. Women with pear-shaped bodies should avoid them, however: Tight jeans will only emphasize your lower half!

Boot Cut

Slightly flared at the legs, this popular cut is flattering for any body type but especially so for us real women with real curves. It gives us two things: thinner hips and longer legs. The slight flare at the ankle draws attention down the leg, thereby creating the appearance of more length and minimizing the curves of the thighs and behind. If you're tall, do wear low-waisted boot cuts. Team your boot cuts with strappy heels or boots, and avoid flat footwear.

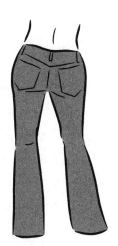

Flared

The extra width of flared jeans helps those with wider hips. However, the wide ankle opening and taper of the leg can look disproportionate on short- or long-torsoed women, so flares work best for tall or long-legged types. Adding heels dresses up the look.

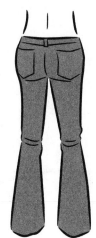

Pockets

Pockets are a great way to create the illusion of lift, form, and fullness—depending on which flatters your shape:

- **Embroidered.** If you have a flat butt, a pocket with texture is good for you. By adding a focal point, the stitching gives the illusion of shape.
- **Angled.** Pockets that are angled make your butt look higher and smaller. Stitching adds more dimension to a flat butt.
- **Drop yoke.** Pockets that are sewn lower on jeans make your butt look more lifted and fit. The pocket hugs your shape for a perkier-looking tush!
- **Button flap.** If you're petite, button-flap pockets are your best choice: The flaps give shape to a less-round butt.

DID YOU KNOW?

In 1999, Levi Strauss was the first jean manufacturer to embrace mass cus-tomization with a program that allows customers to buy a personalized pair of jeans. It made sense for jean manufacturers to adopt the concept, since jeans have to fit more detailed areas of the body. When asked what they like most about their favorite brand of jeans, 69 percent of women said a good fit in the butt was most important to them, followed by comfort at a distant 13 percent.

CHAPTER 5

CHOOSING THE BEST BIKINI

he Myth: Bikinis are only for perfect bodies. Many women mistakenly think that they can hide their physical flaws under a conservative one-piece swimsuit, but remember that even one-piece swimsuits are essentially skin hugging, and flaws may still show in the end. *The Fact:* A woman can look just as good in a bikini that is chosen correctly to flaunt what she has got, and mask what she has not.

A BRIEF HISTORY OF THE BATHING SUIT

The first bathing suits go back to ancient Greece with styles that have little resemblance to the skimpy suits we see today. In ancient times, "coed" swimming was frowned upon. It wasn't until the eighteenth century that men and women could acceptably bathe together. When public bathing began to occur, it more resembled an eighth-grade dance—boys on one side and girls on the other!

The design of the modern bathing suit took over one hundred years to evolve. By the 1800s, more practical swimwear began replacing togas and bathing "gowns." Gone were the restrictive, weighted or woolen suits; instead, swimmers luxuriated in suits that allowed more freedom and movement in the water. Women in particular were starting to become adventurous and discover actual swimming, rather than simply wading in the water.

One-piece blouse-and-pant sets started to appear, and in the nineteenth century the first one-piece suit that didn't require any pins, buttons, zippers or the ubiquitous frilly hem made its debut. With colleges and the Olympics accepting women in the pool, the bathing suit really made some fashion progress. Of course, the volleyball beach bikini was still years and years away. And today, almost anything goes!

GENERAL TIPS

- Choose suits with at least 15 percent spandex to minimize flabby areas.
- Choose your tops and bottoms separately so that you can find the best fit. Separates may sometimes cost a little more, but they're worth the investment!
- Try a size larger for your top, and a size smaller for your bottom.
- If you intend to perform moderate to vigorous activities in your suit, such as swimming or playing beach volleyball, avoid flimsy string bikinis.
- Go for graphic appeal: bright cheerful colors and flirty floral or retro prints rather than plain, simple neutrals.
- If you're unsure about which type and color of bikini to go for, safe bets are halter types in pink tones. Halters are so versatile because they provide enough support for the ample-busted, yet help create the illusion of cleavage for the small-chested. Pink

hues are flattering to almost all skin tones from fair to dark-skinned women, and everything in between.

BEST BIKINI STYLES FOR EACH FIGURE TYPE

Small Breasts

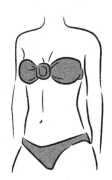

- To create fuller cleavage, wear a padded underwire halter-neck top.
- Printed tops help maximize a small bust.
- Breasts can look bigger with a bandeau top.
- A demi-bra (half-cup) style makes the most of a dainty bust-line.
- Look for a top with adjustable straps that tie behind the neck and around the back so that you can tighten and adjust to help fill out your top line.

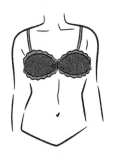

- If you're self-conscious about your small breasts, opt for textured details at the top, such as ruffles and smocking.
- If you're happy with small, perky breasts, you can show them off with those tiny triangle tops!

Big Breasts

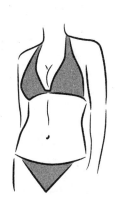

- You may need some extra support. Go for underwire tops to eliminate sagging breasts.
- Halter-top bikinis can be a good choice for bust support while providing sexy cleavage, too.
- Look for styles that are banded around the midriff for that extra lift, with tie-straps around the neck and back to allow for a more personalized fit.

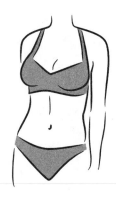

- Wide shoulder straps will be more comfortable than thin spaghetti straps.
- Avoid strapless bandeau tops and flimsy triangle tops that offer minimal coverage. Instead, pick a dark-colored bikini top with a high or square-cut neck.
- Choose a wider-cut bottom to balance out your silhouette.
- Opt for bikini bottoms with a belt, colored band, or drawstring to bring attention to your bottom.

Wide Shoulders

- Play up your lower torso with bikini bottoms that have lots of light color and a printed design.
- Look for decorative elements at the hips—ties, belts, and sashes—to bring attention to your trim bottom.
- Avoid plunging necklines or tiny bikini bottoms that will visually narrow your hips.

Big Hips

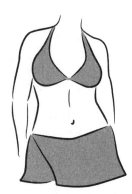

- Wear bikini bottoms that are a shade or two darker than your tops.
- Wear high-cut bikini bottoms that elongate your legs and make your hips and thighs appear slimmer. This cut will also make you look trimmer from behind!
- Avoid horizontal stripes, and opt for vertical prints.
- Miniskirted bikinis are made for you. Just avoid frilly ones that add more volume to the hip area. Pick a smooth, slimming skirt that conceals only where you need it to.
- Draw attention upward with a ruffled or highly decorated top with wider straps to balance out your body proportions.

- Stay away from boy shorts, as well as skimpy or ruffled bottoms. They just add more bulk to your hips.

Short Torso or Legs

- Find a bikini bottom cut high on the thigh. This will make your legs look much longer. If your hips are curvy, this cut will further accentuate your smaller waist and lend a more feminine line.
- Consider wearing a bikini with a plunging neckline to elongate your body.
- Avoid skirted bikinis and boy shorts, which draw the eye downward and can make you look shorter.
- If you're petite, choose bikinis with thin vertical stripes to lengthen your torso.

Long Body

- Boy shorts and ruffled skirts are just the things for your slim hips.
- Avoid vertical stripes, high necklines, and dark solid colors.

Straight Waist

- Try wearing a high-cut bikini bottom, especially with a belted waistline for a more feminine curve.
- Add some illusion of volume at the hips with ruffles, bows, and sashes.

Plus-Sizes

- Go for dark, cool solid colors.
- If you favor prints, choose those with vertical stripes or herringbone V-patterns.

- Sheer sarongs are great as cover-ups—yet so elegant!
- The best styles for you are tankinis that cover the tummy just enough, but are as hip as bikinis.
- Consider a skirted bikini to conceal and divert attention from a too-round bottom.

CHAPTER 6

DECISIONS ON DRESSES

WHERE WE'VE BEEN

Since Coco Chanel introduced it in 1926, the little black dress has become the epitome of timeless fashion. It is the answer to every "What should I wear to . . ." question, from cocktail parties to casinos to class reunions.

A fashion anomaly, the importance of the little black dress never changes, much unlike the trend-crazed fashion industry. It remains the height of chic!

It knows no social, style, or size boundaries. Whether it costs $20 or $2,000, everyone wants to own a little black dress.

WEARING THE LITTLE BLACK DRESS

- Always in style: a sleeveless, kneeish-length (right above, at, or below) sheath.
- Keep your legs bare or in very sheer hose for the dressiest effect.
- Feel free to embellish the look with sparkly earrings, bag, and cover-up: The simple black dress carries accessories well.

Whether you're heading off to a job interview or walking the decks of a cruise ship, the little black dress is a no-fail option. Look for details that flatter your shape (strapless to show off great shoulders; waist details to optimize an hourglass shape), and pick a length anywhere from mini to right below the knee for the most versatile look.

THE TOP DRESS STYLES

- **Empire.** A type of dress or top where the waistline is raised above the natural waistline, sometimes as high as right below the bust. Best on slender-on-top or petite figures, the empire dress creates the illusion of length and camouflages a bottom-heavy figure or thick waist.

- **Strapless.** Strapless frocks can be difficult to pull off, because a too-tight fit can cause armpit or breast bulge, making you appear heavier than you actually are. To ensure that this dress makes your rack look ravishing, choose one that's not too tight and sits comfortably low on your bust to reveal a hint of cleavage. And, of course, a supportive strapless bra is essential; without one, your set might look saggy.

- **Long-sleeved.** A long-sleeved dress can look great, but be sure there isn't a lot of bulky fabric to make you look weighed down.

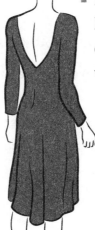

■ **Shirred.** These are so comfortable and versatile, they can be worn with tights and boots in winter. Shirring that comes down to the hips looks great with a belt if your midsection is a problem area. These are very flattering and fun to wear.

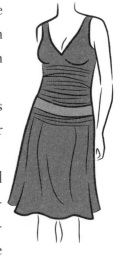

■ **Ruffled.** This is the perfect little black dress with a twist. A sleeveless off-the-shoulder style adds some flare.

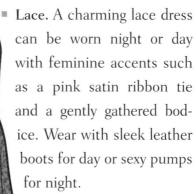

■ **Halter.** This is one of the sexiest formal looks around. Several variations exist, including a knot-front halter and a tie-behind-the-neck look; straps vary in size from spaghetti-width to wide and soft. The halter dress calls extra attention to the upper half of the body, including the face, shoulders, and bustline. This makes it great to help draw unwanted attention away from heavy hips or legs. Skip the necklace with a halter dress: It's just too much going on at the neckline. Opt for long earrings and pulled-up hair for a glamorous touch.

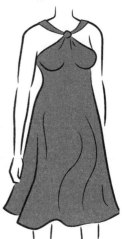

■ **Lace.** A charming lace dress can be worn night or day with feminine accents such as a pink satin ribbon tie and a gently gathered bodice. Wear with sleek leather boots for day or sexy pumps for night.

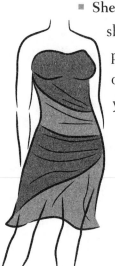

■ **Sheer.** It does take confidence to wear a sheer dress. If you don't have the chutzpah to wear it, then don't. It is one article of clothing that says *Look at me,* and if you're not self-assured, it shows.

CHAPTER 7

HOT HOT HOT HEELS

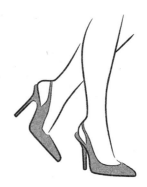

The history of the heel is cloudy, although we know it dates back to pre-Christian times. Egyptian butchers wore high heels to raise them above the carnage, and Mongolian horsemen had heeled boots for gripping their stirrups firmly. The first recorded year heels were worn for vanity was 1533, when Catherine de Médicis brought heels from Florence to Paris for her marriage to the duc d'Orléans. Ladies immediately adopted the style set forth by the French court.

Within the next century, European woman walked on heels five inches and higher, balancing with canes so as not to fall. Because the working class couldn't afford to wear high heels, shoe heights eventually fell. And thereafter they rose or fell according to the fashion.

In the nineteenth century, the high-heeled shoe became the top style to own. Although Europe popularized this new trend, America wasn't far behind. In 1888, the first heel factory in the United States opened; women no longer had to import their shoes from Paris. In the early part of the twentieth century, newly liberated women favored sensible shoes. But in the 1920s, as hemlines rose, legs and feet were suddenly on display and shoes needed to be as beautiful as they were practical. Always fluctuating in and out of style, high heels reached an entirely new level with the advent of the stiletto in the 1950s. And to the chagrin of many a comfortable female, high heels popped up again in fashion magazines in the late '80s and early '90s. Still, whether a woman thinks heels are the height of fashion or the height of pain, if she is a high-heel wearer at all, she usually has at least five pairs in her closet for those occasions when flat shoes just won't do.

CHAPTER 8

SHORTS FOR EVERY WOMAN

Shorts are trendy. Shorts are chic. Wear them with a little jacket or a romantic blouse. Wear them in the city or at your workplace.

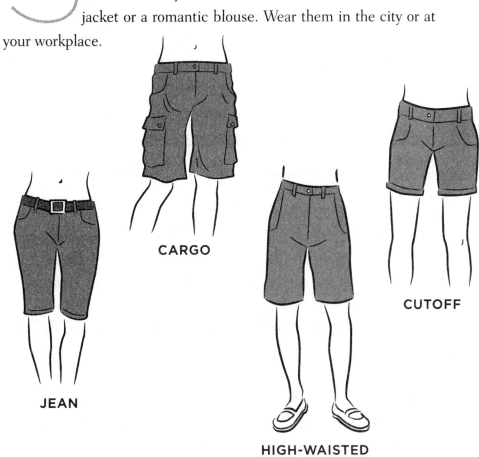

CARGO

JEAN

HIGH-WAISTED

CUTOFF

SHORTS

You'll find them in every warehouse, every boutique, every designer's collection. The "new" shorts are elegant, modern, and good for every occasion. Gone are the times when shorts were considered strictly beachwear. Nowadays you can wear them while shopping, in the office, or to the opening of an art exhibition.

A FEW RULES FOR WEARING SHORTS

- Wear them baggy. Hot pants or tiny shorts are not city-chic. Don't hesitate to buy your shorts one or two sizes bigger than usual. Wear them low on the hip, keep them up with a belt, do whatever you want—but wear them big!
- Go for a specific look, because shorts need a little help. Whether you choose the trendy look or go for the new safari look, make sure it shows. For a sexy effect, wear them with romantic blouses or camisoles, as well as lots of accessories and big belts. If you go for the safari look, complete your outfit with wooden accessories and a fun straw hat.
- Pair knee-length shorts with a classic little jacket and a white blouse. Add a pearl necklace and retro-inspired sunglasses.
- Never wear shorts with stiletto heels. Keep it classy. Go for wedges (very stylish) or Mary Janes (pumps with a fashionable strap across the instep).
- Shorts should never be shorter than you are wide, unless you're in impeccable shape!

When wearing shorts, or anything else, the length should be in proportion to your size, shape, and figure. The hem should hit the shapeliest part of your leg and not be too full or too tight. Showing more leg—when there's leg worth showing—will make you appear taller, as will a shoe with a little lift to it. Wearing an untucked blouse in a complementing color that grazes your figure will also create a longer, leaner visual illusion than would tucking your top in and breaking the line.

If you are going to wear shorts, make sure you pick the right ones. High-waisted gathered shorts make tummies and bums look enormous! If you have short legs, opt for low-rise, flat-fronted longer shorts, which are the most flattering.

A word on short shorts: Go for tiny shorts if you have short legs—an illusion of leg length is best given in high-waisted, midthigh versions that hint of more leg to come. Another tip: Don't buy shorts before you've done the workout. Losing those few pounds and toning up your legs will make a world of difference!

CHAPTER 9

PUTTING IT ALL TOGETHER

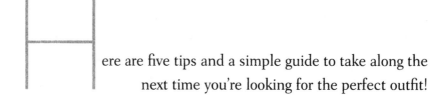

ere are five tips and a simple guide to take along the next time you're looking for the perfect outfit!

FIVE TIPS TO HIDE FIVE EXTRA POUNDS

- **Soft layers.** Keep your layering pieces lightweight, such as tank tops and T-shirts.
- **Add some heels.** High heels with pants give you amazing length and sleekness in your legs.
- **Choose one color.** Dressing in one color helps peel away the pounds. Longer jackets help hide larger bottoms.
- **Sexy blouse.** Sexy tops help soften the look and draw attention to the face.
- **Oversized handbag.** Yes, choosing the right handbag is important and can play tricks on the eye. Choose a shape that flatters (a square shape compliments a rounder figure) and a strap length that doesn't land in the problem area. Never let the bottom of the purse rest on full hips.

TO LOOK TALLER

A single color from shoulders to knee

Narrow and straight silhouettes

Longer garments, rather than shorter

Narrow or straight-legged pants

Shoes with a heel

Plain fabrics, soft, muted colors, plain or small prints, not bulky

TO LOOK SHORTER

Upper and lower garments of contrasting colors

Shoulder, midriff, or hip yokes

Short skirts, wide jackets, boleros

Wide-legged pants

Short skirts, accents at the waistline

Large, bold prints, bulky and textured fabrics

TO LOOK THINNER

Accents near face

Gently fitted styles

Inset or concealed pockets

Vertical lines, long silhouettes

Boat necklines

Pulling your hair up and away from your shoulders

Sheer blouses

Low-riding jeans

No excess fabric

TO LOOK HEAVIER

Accents on heaviest part of body

Bulky and bouffant styles

Patch pockets, cargo pants

Curved, horizontal, or diagonal lines

WHAT TO KEEP, WHAT TO TOSS

Wardrobe planning is an important step when determining what to wear. You should conduct a wardrobe inventory to see what exactly you own, what you like, what needs to be thrown out, and what you need to add. Ask yourself a few questions before making any decisions:

- *Does it flatter my shape?*
- *Does the fit work with my body type?*
- *Has this been in my closet for the past four years, unworn?*
- *Do I feel like a million bucks when I wear it?*

When you are ready to add garments to your wardrobe, consider the following ways to increase the usefulness of the clothing you buy and the existing items in your closet:

- Basic or classic styles last for several years.
- Accessories harmonize better with simple classic lines and versatile textures in "quiet" colors.
- Less expensive accessories can be changed to make an outfit look different or new.
- Choose separates based on the same color scheme. These can be mixed or matched to create different outfits and greater variety.
- Spend less money on fad clothing, more on classic pieces that will last for several years.
- Check out many different resources when purchasing clothing: department stores, discount outlets, consignment shops, garage sales, and secondhand stores. You will not believe the finds!

PART II

Working It All Out!

CHAPTER 10

WHAT TO EXPECT WHEN YOU'RE EXPECTING (NOT A BABY!)

REASONABLE WORKOUT EXPECTATIONS

You probably bought this book because you want to start working out. If you have any sense, you should know that if you want to fit into that gorgeous cocktail dress next month, starving yourself is not the answer. Exercise is the key, and in addition to being healthful, it can even be fun.

How Physically Fit Are You?

Before beginning any exercise program, it is extremely important to consult with your family physician. After receiving medical clearance, you should assess your fitness level. A fitness assessment consists of determining your present condition in a number of areas, including heart rate, blood pressure, body weight, body fat percentage, measurements, flexibility, lean body weight, and more. Once you know the results of your fitness assessment, it becomes easier to determine your fitness goals. If you don't know where you are to start with, you won't know where you want to go. Another reason to have assessments done on a regular basis is to provide motivation when you see progress from one to the next. By comparing these numbers, you can determine what parts of your training program are working and what might need to be tweaked or changed.

GOALS: KEEP IT SIMPLE

Before you can decide on your goals, you must determine reasonable expectations. Write these down and look at this list from time to time. Remember, the key word is *reasonable*! Do you want to tone your arms? Tighten your bum? These are reasonable thoughts, reachable goals. If you want to look like Angelina Jolie in two weeks . . . fahgeddaboutit. Besides, this is about looking your best in the body you have, and in the clothes you love.

In the short term, you must create your fitness goals on a day-by-day basis. Eating healthfully and exercising are the first steps toward achieving your fitness goals. The day-by-day approach allows you to maintain discipline and focus. The next step is to incorporate a healthy lifestyle into a longer period of time—say, one or two weeks. It's really useful during this period to keep track of your progress with a calendar or notebook. This gives you quick visual feedback on your progress. It's good to give yourself tangible, positive reinforcement.

A longer-term goal consists of following your routine for an extended period of time, such as six to eight weeks. You can really make a noticeable difference in how you look and feel over this longer time period. When committing yourself to a long-term goal, it's wise to reward yourself in some way each week. Enjoy your favorite ice cream (only one scoop!) or, if you prefer, buy that pair of shoes you've been eyeing. Whatever your reward, know that it can help you stick with your long-term program, especially when you hit the wall and feel like you can't go on. Which brings us to the next crucial step in getting your new bod.

MOTIVATING YOURSELF TO BUFF UP

We all know that exercise is good for us: It helps reduce the risk of heart disease, assists with weight management, and can control cholesterol, diabetes, and high blood pressure. Exercise boosts energy levels and helps manage stress. Studies show that it can extend our lives and improve our quality of life, too. Moreover, according to the *Surgeon General's Report on Physical Activity and Health,* higher levels of regular physical activity are associated with lower mortality rates for both older and younger adults. Even those who are moderately active on a regular basis have lower rates of mortality than those who are least active.

So why are fewer than half of Americans leading a moderately active lifestyle? In a recent study, 16,890 women and men eighteen years old and above were asked about their leisure-time physical activities. Only 38 percent met the surgeon general's guideline of thirty minutes of moderate physical activity most, if not all, days of the week. Most alarming, however, is that *women,* ethnic minorities, adults with lower educational attainment, and older adults were least active. Furthermore, according to this same report about 25 percent of adults took part in no physical activity at all in their leisure time.

FITTING EXERCISE IN

Too busy to exercise? Incorporate it into your day! You've probably heard of some of the ways you can do that: Park farther away from the entrance to your office or the shopping mall. Take the stairs instead of the elevator. Engage in play with your kids or the dog.

Too tired to exercise? Get out of the habit of rushing everywhere and take time to take care of your body. If the store is a few blocks away and you only need an item or two, walk instead of driving. Rather than go to the movies on a beautiful Saturday afternoon, go to the zoo, stroll through an art gallery, or go for a hike. Rushing everywhere puts unnecessary stress on your mind and body. Get your heart pumping for another reason. Be interactive instead of inactive.

A DOZEN BUFF TIPS

- Make time for exercise. Get up half an hour earlier, walk during lunch, or turn off the television in the evening.
- Make it fun. Choose activities that you enjoy. Gardening and walking are the two most popular forms of exercise among women.
- Make sure you have a variety of activities to choose from so that you don't get bored and drop your exercise program.
- Be creative. Instead of calling a friend, arrange to get together for a walk-and-talk once or twice a week.
- Involve your family. Take the kids along for walks and bike rides. Spend quality time with your partner while enjoying an outdoor activity.
- Set fitness goals. Commit to walking or running a certain distance in one month, three months, or six months. Work on increasing the number of laps you swim each day.
- Train for an event—a walkathon, bike-athon, or triathlon. If you need support, get a friend to join you. The event can also be that twenty-year high school reunion coming up!
- Give yourself a reward for your fitness accomplishments.
- Find a convenient time and place for your exercise. Schedule this time and honor it. If you are unable to exercise for some reason, make it up as soon as possible. This is the biggest reason why we backslide. We miss one,

then two workouts, and before we know it, it's been two weeks, and who wants to start over?

- Start slowly and work up to exercising three to five times a week for thirty to sixty minutes.

- The more often you work out, the less time you have to set aside for it. For example, working out three times a week for sixty minutes requires a bigger time commitment than working out five times a week for thirty minutes. If you're really pressed for time, break the thirty-minute session into two fifteen-minute segments or three ten-minute segments.

- Once you've made regular exercise part of your lifestyle, don't stop there. Greater health benefits can be obtained by engaging in physical activity of a more vigorous intensity or of longer duration. Moreover, recent recommendations from experts suggest that endurance activity should be supplemented with strength-developing exercises at least twice per week for adults.

FITNESS ON THE ROAD

Whether you travel often or only occasionally, disruptions in your exercise routine can seriously derail it. And if your exercise routine disappears, your hard-earned fitness and strength gains can leave you within weeks. But all is not lost. A little planning and effort can give you a fitness plan for almost any out-of-town trip.

Road-Trip Reasoning

Begin your travel plan by reducing expectations when away from home. Sure, you've been training hard to tone your muscles, and you're eager to keep the momentum going. But is this reasonable when on the road?

If you're well rested and blessed with sufficient facilities and time, go for it. For some travelers, hotel health clubs and free evenings provide them with ideal opportunities to boost their fitness. Also, strive to eat healthfully by focusing on wise food selections. You can even come back home a bit healthier than when you left!

Most business travelers, though, will be shortchanged somewhere along the line on opportunities to exercise, so it's best to anticipate this by not expecting too much of yourself. Maintaining strength and fitness is much easier than building it. When you're out of town, therefore, concentrate on maintaining your gains through modest training. As little as one or two moderate workouts a week can maintain your fitness level.

If you're on the road, this may be a good time to switch to an alternative mode of exercise. This may revitalize your body, giving you more energy for training than you had before leaving. The energy you get from comfortable, moderate exercise may even boost your productivity during your time away.

Road-Trip Tips

Here are some other on-the-road exercise tips to keep in mind. Use whatever ideas fit your style and schedule, or think up your own ways to stay active while traveling.

- **Lay the groundwork.** Plan ahead when choosing accommodations. Choose hotels with good fitness facilities. Call before booking to make sure you'll have access to what you need. If there's no gym available at your hotel, inquire as to the nearest facilities.

- **Do something.** Commit to doing some form of exercise. When it comes to your health, consistency is the key. Don't give up on exercise just because you can't get out for your three-mile run. Be flexible and take a walk instead. As the ad says, "Just do it!"

- **Hit the ground running.** Set the tone for your trip by exercising as soon as you can after arriving at your destination. Working out right away affirms your commitment, helps relieve the stress and fatigue of traveling, aids in adjusting to jet lag, and eliminates the chance that later events will sidetrack your exercise program for the whole trip.

- **Pencil in exercise.** If you can't get in a bout of exercise immediately, schedule workout time by blocking out an hour in your daily planner.

- **Find fitness snippets.** If you're strapped for time, seek exercise opportunities in bits and pieces. Avoid escalators and climb the stairs. Fast-walk in the hotel hallways. If distance allows, walk to an appointment. When confronted with a layover, stroll the terminal instead of reading the paper.

- **Discover fun.** Build some fun into your exercise routine. Ask the hotel concierge to help you map out a scenic walking or jogging tour. Walking, or even jogging, through a city can give you an up-close experience that can't be matched on a tour bus. But make sure you know where you're going and avoid areas where being a pedestrian could make you a target.

- **Protect your joints.** Be careful when running. If you must jog on sidewalks, know that cement is hard on hip and leg joints. Reduce your speed and distance.

- **Gear up.** Pack gear that will prepare you for a variety of exercise opportunities. Shoes designed for your specific activity are a must. Take exercise clothes suitable for indoor and outdoor conditions, and pack a swimsuit.

■ **Try suite sweat.** Don't underestimate the value of exercising in your room. Old standards such as push-ups, lunges, crunches, and jumping jacks require only your energy and a small space. Plan ahead by designing a fifteen- to twenty-minute routine that keeps you moving.

■ **Pack a gym.** Bring your own mini-gym. You can get a good work-out with portable rubber exercise tubing, handgrips, plastic dumbbells that fill with water, a jump rope, or videos that guide you in fitness, yoga, or stretching routines. And if appropriate, don't forget sports equipment—a tennis or racquetball racket, golf clubs, what have you.

■ **Tune in.** Check the TV for exercise programs. The local channel listings might offer good fitness shows that you can exercise along with.

CHAPTER 11

CREATING YOUR OWN HOME BUFF GYM

Working out at home is just easier! Plus, you can't use logistics as an excuse for not working out. The number one excuse people give for skipping workouts is not having time to go to the gym. When you're really busy or if you're tired, it's harder to motivate yourself when you're looking at travel time and workout time versus just getting straight down to business. This is especially true for those new moms out there. But having a gym in your own home makes things so much easier for everyone. The biggest challenge is making a small space feel roomy enough to work out in. Here are some of the benefits of working out at home:

- You can't talk yourself out of it in the time it takes you to put on your workout clothes and get to your car.
- No snowstorm, hurricane, or other act of God that closes the roads will prevent you from getting there.
- You can wear what you woke up in (and look like you just woke up!).
- The sweat on the exercise mat is yours.
- No lines. You don't have to share equipment with some chemically enhanced musclehead.

- No embarrassment! So what if you're doing bicep curls with five-pound dumbbells?
- No membership fees.
- No annoying aspiring models in view.
- You can play your own music . . . as loud as you want.
- No matter how small your space is, you can cheaply and effectively outfit your house or apartment with a suitable workout area. Though prices and styles depend on the supplier, basic strength-training equipment is comparable. I tell all of my clients that a $25 set of five-pound dumbbells weighs the same as a $15 set of five-pound dumbbells.

There is really zero difference between a gym membership and a home gym if your goal is to see fitness results. Your body doesn't know the difference between a high-tech gym and your basement! Results are all up to you.

Before you start making a list of equipment to buy, take a look around your house to see what you can use:

- If your coffee table is sturdy and wide enough, it can be a great bench and step. Make sure it's at least twelve to twenty inches wide and sturdy enough to hold your weight.
- An ottoman is great for tricep dips and step-ups.
- Stairs can give you a good cardio warm-up. Climb a few flights before your workout and you're ready to go!
- Water bottles, buckets (don't forget to fill them!), and canned vegetables all make great dumbbells for the beginner.

WHAT TO BUY FOR YOUR BUFF GYM

So you're ready to go to your local sporting goods store to buy some equipment. Before you spend a dime, you should ask yourself a few questions. First: *What is my goal?* Although this book will give you very specific workouts for very specific goals, you may have other fitness dreams that you want to combine with these workouts. For example, you may have a certain cardiovascular goal you want to reach. With that said, you must think about that part of your workout and what you like to do (see the next chapter, "Don't Forget the Cardio"). Second: *Do I have enough space to set up an adequate workout area?* If you live in a tiny apartment, push the couch and TV against the wall so you can move freely. If you plan on using videos for the cardiovascular component of the workout, make sure you read the description of the video carefully in case you need to buy any additional equipment. *Let's get started!*

Dumbbells

Dumbbells are among the most practical purchases you can make, because they're so versatile. They come in various shapes, sizes, and colors. They also come in various prices. If more expensive dumbbells will make you use them more, go for it! But the less expensive and less flashy ones do the same job. Do, however, stay away from dumbbells filled with sand. After a while, with use, you may find the sand in your eyes. Dumbbells can be bought at most department stores, sporting goods stores, specialty shops, or even yard sales. A specialty shop may have more of a selection, but they will probably be more expensive.

Depending on your level of strength, start off with a few sets of dumbbells, increasing in weight. For women who are beginners and intermediates, I recommend dumbbells weighing three, five, eight, ten, twelve, and fifteen pounds. That should be fine to start. Once you become more advanced, you can add to your collection. If you do accumulate a lot of dumbbells over time, a rack is a great way to store them. If you have limited space and time, there are such things as adjustable dumbbells. The kit usually contains two small bars and a number of plates that you clip on with collars.

Fitness Ball

A fitness ball is an excellent addition to your home gym. Once used only by physical therapy patients in rehabilitation, they can now be found in almost every gym. Fitness balls work on the concept of core strength and balance. The core muscle groups are the abdominals and the muscles of the lower back, hips, and spine. Most people have incredibly weak core muscle strength. Using the fitness ball also enables you to enhance your balance and coordination. These balls come in all colors and sizes and range in price from about $20 to $40, depending on durability. Before buying a cheaper brand, make sure that it's an anti-bust ball.

BALL SIZES

The recommended ball size is one that allows you to bend your knees at a ninety-degree angle. When sitting on the ball with your feet flat on the floor, your ankles should be directly under your knees in a straight line.

- If you're four foot eight to five foot three in height, get a fifty-five-centimeter ball.
- If your height is five foot four to six feet, look for a sixty-five-centimeter model.
- Those six feet and taller need a seventy-five-centimeter ball.

You can use a larger ball if:

- Your legs are longer.
- You're overweight.
- You're using a ball only for stretching.

You can use a smaller ball if:

- You have shorter legs.
- You're at the lower end of the height range.

Mat

A stretching mat is a good investment, especially if your workout surface is hard. A mat is great for doing abdominal exercises and any other exercises that require you to be on the floor. It also prevents the fitness ball, your feet, and your hands from slipping and sliding when you're performing certain exercises. A decent mat should run the length from your head to your butt, and be thick enough to allow comfort on a hard surface. It can run you anywhere from $15 to $35.

Bench

If you decide to purchase a bench (many of the exercises I outline can be done on a bench or fitness ball), go for an adjustable incline bench—one that adjusts from a flat position all the way up to vertical. A good bench may run you around $100. Check your local newspaper or eBay for a secondhand model.

Step

A step is more expensive (a good one goes for around $85 or so), but you can use it for everything from step aerobics to a weight bench to a plant holder (although I don't recommend it for your gardening . . .).

Mirror

I really think this is a crucial piece of equipment for your home gym. The purpose of a mirror is not simply to check yourself out and see if your hair is in place! You need a mirror to check your form, especially when you're doing free-weight exercises. Make sure you get one long enough so you can see your whole body while performing an exercise.

Sneakers, Socks, and Workout Clothes

I know this may be obvious, but a good pair of sneakers is a must when working out. Few things are more inspiring for your fitness regimen than a new pair of running or walking shoes. When your energy, excitement, or motivation dips, a new pair of kicks can get you moving again. By *good* pair, I don't mean the sneakers with heels or Velcro that offer little support. Believe it or not, I often train people who show up with sandals on. If you drop a weight wearing sandals, look out, poor toes! If you wear shoes without rubber soles, you may do a lot of slipping and sliding during your workout.

Equally as important as your shoes is your choice of socks. Be sure that when you go to try on shoes, you wear the socks you'll be working out in. Choose Thorlos or any socks made of CoolMax, rather than standard cotton. Your feet will be much more comfortable, drier, and are more likely to stay blister-free in this fabric.

Proper clothing is definitely necessary while working out as well. Invest in a couple of tops and bottoms that allow your skin to breathe and cool off while you exercise. Jeans and any bulky clothing are a bad idea; it's also hard to check out your form with clothes that hide your body. Treat yourself! Having cool, funky workout clothes is a great motivator.

Workout Gloves

Perhaps I'm getting carried away, but I do think gloves are a good investment if you're the sensitive-hand type. Weight-lifting gloves have padded palms, and the tops of the fingers are cut off. They're good at preventing calluses and slippage. Plus, you will look and feel like the real deal!

Water Bottle

When exercising at home, don't get distracted by running into the kitchen every time you want water. Have a water bottle nearby at all times; you'll tend to drink more.

iPod, MP3 Player, or Radio

The great thing about working out at home is, you get to choose the music to keep you going!

Training Log

Having a log is another great motivator. It also enables you to see your progress (or lack thereof) over a period of time. Keep a separate log for each buff workout!

SAMPLE DAILY WORKOUT LOG

Day of Week: Date:

Goals: Buff in a Tank Top

Cardiovascular Activity: Time:

Strength-Training Exercise	Weight	Sets	Reps
1.			
2.			
3.			
4.			
5.			

Notes:

Other Stuff

- **Jump rope.** Jumping rope makes a perfect cardio activity in a pinch or if you're on the road and can't find your favorite machine.
- **Resistance band.** This is also a good fitness traveler when you can't pack your dumbbells.
- **Fitness DVDs.** Good for motivation, easy to carry, and the music is always good!

CHAPTER 12

DON'T FORGET THE CARDIO

The mission of this book is to get you started on a weight-training program that can put you on your way to feeling good, no matter what you're wearing! All good strength-training workouts should be supplemented with three to four cardio sessions per week. This cardiovascular section is to remind you why you need to combine your weight training with some kind of activity that raises your heart rate. I'm not suggesting that you buy a treadmill or elliptical machine. I just want you to be aware of some of the many cardio options you can incorporate into your life.

A FEW FACTS

Of my clients, 99.99 percent want to tone up and build some muscle—but also to "lose a few pounds." Strength training alone is not going to make that happen. Muscles are nice, but they'll remain hidden if a layer of fat covers them up. The most effective way to lose fat is by having a plan that balances strength training, aerobic exercise, and a good diet. The key word is *balance,* a fitness concept I stress with my clients.

Aerobic exercise includes any type of activity that raises your heart rate and allows you to burn a lot of calories in a short period of time. Popular aerobic activities include power walking, jogging, biking, and swimming. But your choices are not limited to just these. Jumping rope, climbing stairs, jumping jacks—any repetitive activity that involves your large muscle groups and lasts longer than a minute and a half counts.

Cardiovascular exercise also strengthens your heart and lungs. Having a strong heart means that your heart beats fewer times per minute to pump the same amount of blood. Over the course of a day, this can really add up. Over the course of ten years, you've just saved billions of heartbeats! Having strong lungs means you're getting more oxygen per breath, which means more stamina during the day. You will notice with time, if you're consistent with your workouts, that your stamina improves and you're able to get through your workouts and your day with more energy.

FREQUENTLY ASKED CARDIO QUESTIONS

How Many Days a Week Should I Do Cardio?

At least four days per week. Even if you don't have a weight-loss goal, you should still want to maintain good health and reduce your risk of heart and lung disease, high blood pressure, and other serious conditions. Beginners should start with twenty minutes per day, while the more advanced can shoot for thirty to forty-five minutes, four to five days per week. Most of my clients have a hard time finding thirty to forty-five consecutive minutes, four times per week. It's okay to string a workout together, meaning three ten-minute workouts during the day. But in order to really see a difference in your stamina and weight, you will need to include longer aerobic workouts during the week.

How Hard Should I Work Out?

The second component of cardiovascular exercise—after frequency—is duration, which refers to the time you spend exercising. The cardiovascular session, not including the warm-up and cool-down, should range from twenty to sixty minutes to gain significant cardiorespiratory and fat-burning benefits. Each time you do your cardiovascular exercise, try to do twenty minutes or more. Of course, the longer you go, the more calories and fat you'll burn and the better you'll condition your cardiovascular system. All beginners, especially those who are out of shape, should take a very conservative approach and train at relatively low intensities (50 to 70 percent of your maximum heart rate) for ten to twenty-five minutes. As you get into better shape, you can gradually increase the amount of time you exercise.

It's important that you gradually increase the duration *before* you increase the intensity. That is, when beginning a walking program (for example), be more concerned with increasing the number of minutes of the exercise session before you increase your speed or take on hilly terrain.

DID YOU KNOW?

America is the fattest country in the world, and we spent more than $33 billion last year alone on diet and weight-loss products. According to a recent study, less than 10 percent of the population exercises three or more times a week at a level vigorous enough to improve cardiovascular fitness.

How Quickly Will I See Results?

Most people swear they see and feel a difference after a couple of workouts! That may be true emotionally, but it will take several weeks of consistent aerobic workouts to make a real difference in your stamina and energy level. Instant gratification is what most people want when starting an exercise plan. Stay patient and consistent!

What Cardio Activity Is the Best?

What activity do you like? Well then, that's the best! Find something you enjoy; the number one reason people fall off the fitness wagon is because they get bored or they hate what they're doing. Cross-training, or the combination of activities during one workout, not only will prevent boredom, but will also allow your body to burn calories more efficiently and keep your heart and lungs strong. For example, you could bike for ten minutes at a good intensity, then jog for the remaining twenty minutes. "Tricking" your body and doing many activities at varying intensities is the best way to go! Stretching, cardiovascular activities, and strength training are the three elements of a fitness routine that will yield positive results.

TARGET HEART RATE

To get the most out of your workout, you should frequently check your pulse and get into your target heart rate zone.

Wearing a heart rate monitor is an easy, accurate method of checking your heart rate . . . but if you don't have a monitor, there's another easy way to get the same information.

The easiest place to feel your own heartbeat is the carotid artery. Place your index finger on the side of your neck between the middle

WORKING IT ALL OUT!

of your collarbone and your jawline. (You can also use the radial artery on the underside of your wrist.) You can count the beats for a full sixty seconds, or count for six seconds and add a zero at the end. If you felt your heart beat 14 times in six seconds, for example, the total would be 140 for a full minute. Counting for only six seconds is a convenient method, though of course it's more accurate to count for the full sixty. You can also use several variations on this method: thirty seconds times two, or fifteen seconds times four, or the like. The longer you count, the more accurate your reading. Whatever you choose, be consistent in your method.

To determine your target training zone, take your resting pulse three mornings in a row, just after waking up. Add all of them together and divide by three to get the average. Let's say your average is sixty beats per minute.

(220)−(your age) = MaxHR

(MaxHR)−(resting heart rate) = HRR (heart rate recovery)

(HRR) × (60% to 80%) = training range %

(training range %) + (resting heart rate) = (your target training zone)

So:

220−35 = 185 (MaxHR)

185−60 = 125 (HRR)

125 × 0.6 = 75 (60% training percentage)

125 × 0.8 = 100 (80% training percentage)

75 + 60 = 135 (target training zone, in beats per minute)

100 + 60 = 160 (target training zone, in beats per minute)

Your target training zone, in beats per minute, is between 135 and 160. Of course, to get a fifteen-second target, simply divide each number by four. That would be thirty-four to forty beats over fifteen seconds. When counting beats, start with the first beat as zero: 0–1–2–3–4 . . . 38–39–40.

Training Zones

- **Healthy heart zone (warm-up):** 50 to 60 percent of maximum heart rate. This is the easiest zone and probably the best one for people just starting a fitness program. It can also be used as a warm-up for more serious exercisers. This zone has been shown to help decrease body fat, blood pressure, and cholesterol. It also decreases the risk of degenerative diseases and has a low risk of injury. Eighty-five percent of calories burned in this zone are fats!

- **Fitness zone (fat burning):** 60 to 70 percent of maximum heart rate. This zone provides the same benefits as the healthy heart zone, but is more intense and burns more total calories. The percent of fat calories burned is still 85.

- **Aerobic zone (endurance training):** 70 to 80 percent of maximum heart rate. The aerobic zone will improve your cardiovascular and respiratory system *and* increase the size and strength of your heart. This is the preferred zone if you're training for an endurance event. More calories are burned, with 50 percent of them from fat.

- **Anaerobic zone (performance training):** 80 to 90 percent of maximum heart rate. The benefits of this zone include an improved VO_2 maximum (the highest amount of oxygen you can consume during exercise) and thus an improved cardiorespiratory system, along with a higher lactate tolerance, which means your endurance will improve and you'll be able to fight fatigue better. This is a high-intensity zone, burning more calories, 15 percent of them from fat.

- **Red line (maximum effort):** 90 to 100 percent of maximum heart rate. Although this zone burns the greatest number of calories, it is very intense. Most people can stay in this zone only for short periods. You should train here only if you're in very good shape and have been cleared by a physician to do so.

You should be able to carry on a conversation during your workout. If you're breathless or can't talk, you're working too hard! Slow down. Also, keep in mind that dizziness and light-headedness are *not* good signs. If you experience these, you are overexerting yourself and should stop!

THE WARM-UP

Yes, everyone needs to warm up. A warm-up may consist of many different activities and exercises, but you need to do something that warms up your body. Five to seven minutes should be enough time to get your muscles ready for action.

POPULAR CARDIO OPTIONS

Power Walking

I can't think of an easier way to get in a fast cardio workout. Lace up your sneakers and walk around your local park, school track, or block for thirty minutes. Drive your elbow back with each step for an added calorie-burning boost.

Some of the benefits of walking are:

- It burns calories.
- It strengthens your back muscles.
- It slims your waist.
- It is easy on your joints.
- It strengthens your bones.
- It can lower your blood pressure.
- It allows you time with family and friends.
- It shapes and tones your legs and butt.
- It cuts your cholesterol.
- It can reduce your risk of heart disease, diabetes, and more.
- It can reduce stress.
- It helps you sleep better.
- It improves your mood and outlook on life.
- It can be done almost anywhere.
- It requires no equipment.
- It's free!

Jogging

You see joggers everywhere! If you're new to jogging, start with power walking for your first couple of weeks. Gradually incorporate jogging with a run-for-one-minute, walk-for-three-minutes format. If you're not an outdoor jogger, treadmills are just as effective. If you decide to power walk, drive your elbows back as you walk. If you run at less than four and a half miles per hour, you'll burn fewer calories than walking at that pace. Also, try not to run with short steps; lengthen your stride and speed up slightly. Once you hit your running stride (over four and a half miles per hour), don't cheat by taking short steps. Short steps slow you down, thereby burning fewer calories. If calorie burning is your goal, add a 3 to 5 percent incline. You may not feel much of a difference, but you'll see an increase in calories expended. If you're a walker, you'll have a tough time going faster, but you *can* work harder by using the incline feature.

Biking

Whether you're on a stationary or a road bike, the way to maximize your workout is *not* to pedal like a maniac; it's to add resistance and slow your speed. Aim to keep a cadence of seventy to eighty revolutions per minute (rpms). Once you hit one hundred rpms, caloric expenditure goes down. When you're pedaling that fast, you're probably not using enough resistance to challenge yourself.

You also want to make sure the seat positioning is correct on a stationary bike. Whether you're on a recumbent or an upright bike, adjust the seat so your knee has a slight bend when your leg is fully extended. On an upright bike, try not to sit up tall and hold the front of the handlebars. Instead, round over the handlebars to take the pressure off your lower back and increase circulation in your legs.

A question I'm frequently asked is, "Which burns more calories: the upright or recumbent bike?" If you use the same exact workload—say, level 8 on both machines—you'll burn 15 to 25 percent more calories on the upright bike. On an upright bike, you're lifting your legs against gravity, which requires more energy. On a recumbent bike, you've got a nice comfy seat with back support and you're pushing horizontally. The pedaling motion is more efficient but you're burning fewer calories.

Elliptical Machine

You've probably noticed folks in your local gym going as fast as they can on the elliptical, arms and legs a blur. Instead of increasing the speed to push yourself harder, add resistance and/or change the ramp position. Speed will help you burn calories, but only to a point. Once you begin moving out of control, you're unable to work harder and you burn fewer calories. Resistance does the job better, while different ramp sections allow you to challenge different muscle groups for more of an overall workout.

Stair Climbing

The stair climber is the most frequently misused machine on the market. It's important to keep good form on the StairMaster. Keep your body upright, with your hands lightly touching the handles. Leaning heavily on the handlebars so you can go faster only decreases how hard your legs must work, cutting the calories expended. Better yet, try not touching the handles at all and pumping your arms. Or alternate between holding on and letting go for a minute at a time. It's also important to remember to take deep steps, not shallow, choppy ones. Deeper steps mean larger muscle groups are engaged, so you burn more calories.

Swimming

Check out your local Y or gym for another great cardio option. Many people prefer to swim, because it has less impact on the knees.

CHAPTER 13

GETTING STARTED

You're almost ready to get started. In the pages ahead, you will learn exercises that will help you look ripped in a tank top, get your best buns for those favorite jeans of yours, be slim and sleek in a little black dress, attain more "lift" in stiletto heels, enjoy a better body for that skimpy bikini, and get some show-offy legs with the shorts workout. Here are a few tips to remember:

- Begin with five to ten minutes of cardio to warm up.
- Beginners: As a rule of thumb, do 1 or 2 sets of 10–12 reps of each exercise, using light weights. My recommendations follow each exercise.
- Intermediate/Advanced: Do 3 or more sets of 8–12 reps, using enough weight so that you can complete only the desired number of reps.
- Rest at least one day between workouts.
- Perform each rep slowly by counting to three during each part of the motion.
- After your workout, be sure to stretch.

SEQUENCE OF EXERCISES

Make sure you choose at least one exercise for each major muscle group. The muscles to work include:

- Chest (little black dress)
- Back (little black dress, tank top)
- Shoulders (tank top, little black dress)
- Biceps (tank top)
- Triceps (tank top)
- Quadriceps (shorts)
- Hamstrings and glutes (jeans)
- Abdominals (bikini)

If you leave any muscle group out, this could cause an imbalance in your muscles and possibly lead to injuries.

Most experts recommend starting with your larger muscle groups and proceeding to the smaller muscle groups. The most demanding exercises are those performed by your large muscle groups, and you will need your smaller muscles to get the most out of these exercises. For example, in a chest press, your shoulders and triceps are used to stabilize your arms. You want strong shoulders and triceps so you don't drop the weight on your chest. The bonus? By the time you get to your shoulder and triceps exercises, your muscles will be warmed up and ready to go. This isn't written in stone, however, so do what works for you. In addition, you don't necessarily need to do as many sets with your smaller muscle groups, since they're used so much in other exercises.

HOW MUCH WEIGHT TO USE

The easiest way to determine how much weight you should use on each lift is to guess.

Pick up a light weight and do a warm-up set of the exercise of your choice, aiming for about 10–12 repetitions. Try starting with a five-pound dumbbell.

For set 2, increase your weight by five or more pounds and perform your goal number of repetitions. If you can do more than your desired number of reps, add more weight for your third set.

In general, you should be lifting just enough weight so that you can do *only* the desired number of reps. You should be struggling by the last rep, but still able to finish it with good form. It may take a while to find the right amount of weight for each exercise. You can use heavier weights with larger muscle groups such as chest, back, and legs. You'll need smaller weights for the shoulders and arms.

HOW MANY REPS/SETS TO DO

Now that you've figured out how much weight to use for your chosen exercises, what about the number of sets and repetitions? Your decision should be based on your goals. The American College of Sports Medicine recommends 8–12 reps for muscular strength and 10–15 reps for muscular endurance. It also recommends at least 1 set of each exercise to fatigue, although you'll find that most people perform about 3 sets of each exercise. In general:

- **For fat loss.** Do 10–12 reps using enough weight that you can complete *only* the desired reps, and 1–3 sets (1 for beginners, 2–3 for intermediate and advanced exercisers). Rest for thirty seconds to one minute between sets, and at least one day between workout sessions.

- **For muscle gain.** Do 6–8 reps using enough weight that you can complete *only* the desired reps, and 3 or more sets, resting for a minute or two between sets and three or more days between sessions.

For beginners, give yourself several weeks of conditioning before going to the next level.

HOW LONG TO REST BETWEEN EXERCISES/WORKOUT SESSIONS

Again, this will depend on your goal. Higher-intensity exercise (such as when lifting heavy weights) requires a longer rest. When using lighter weight and more repetitions, it takes between thirty seconds and one minute for your muscles to rest.

The American College of Sports Medicine recommends training each muscle group two to three times a week. But the number of times you lift each week will depend on your training method. In order for muscles to repair and grow, you'll need about forty-eight hours of rest between workout sessions. If you're training at a high intensity, take a longer rest.

STRETCHING AND WARMING UP TO GET BUFF

Flexibility is one of the key components of a balanced fitness program. Without flexibility training (stretching), you're missing an important part of overall health. Flexibility prevents injury, increases range of motion, promotes relaxation, improves performance and posture, reduces stress, and keeps your body feeling loose and agile. Although there is still some controversy over which flexibility exercises are the best and how often you should stretch, most fitness professionals agree that the principles and guidelines of flexibility training that are about to be discussed are the safest and most effective.

Use Static Stretching

Static stretching involves a slow, gradual, and controlled lengthening of a muscle through the full range of motion, held for fifteen to thirty seconds in the farthest comfortable (without pain) position. This is the first and most important stretching principle. I like to use the term *mild discomfort*.

Daily stretching is best, and when done before, during, and after exercise sessions. Frequent stretching will help you avoid muscular imbalances, knots, tightness, and muscle soreness created by daily activities and exercise.

Always Warm Up Before Stretching

A warm muscle is much more easily stretched than a cold one. Never stretch a cold muscle; always warm up first to get blood circulating throughout the body and into the muscles. A warm-up should be a slow, rhythmic exercise of larger muscle groups done before an activity. Riding a bicycle or walking works well. This provides the body with a period of adjustment between rest and the activity. The warm-up should last five to ten minutes and should be similar to the activity that you are about to do, but at a much lower intensity. A good warm-up for strength training could include jumping jacks for five minutes, jumping rope, or a short run around the block. Once you have warmed up at a low intensity for five to ten minutes and have gotten your muscles warm, you can now stretch.

Stretch Before and After Exercise

I recommend stretching both before and after exercise, but for different reasons. Stretching before an activity (after the warm-up) improves dynamic flexibility and reduces the chance of injury. Stretching after exercise ensures muscle relaxation, facilitating normal resting length, circulation to joint and tissue structures, and removal of unwanted waste products, thus reducing muscle soreness and stiffness. Body temperature is highest right after the cardiovascular exercise program and/or after strength training. In order to achieve maximum results in range of motion and other benefits, I highly recommend that you do static stretching at this point in your workout, just after your cardiovascular program and during or after your strength-training program.

Stretch Between Strength-Training Sets

Both strength training and flexibility training are so important for everyone. Those of you who have a hard time finding time to incorporate a strength-training program into your lifestyle can combine your stretching with your strength-training program. If you have had any experience in strength training, you know that for each exercise for each muscle group you train, you have a certain number of sets, usually 1–4. Between each set, you need to rest and let your muscle recover before going on to the next set. Well, what better use of your resting time than to stretch the specific muscle you're currently training? Think about it: You've just done a set of 10 reps of squats. Now you have to rest, usually for thirty to forty-five seconds, before going on to the next set. This is a great time to stretch your legs—they're already warm, and you have time before you start your next set.

Stretch Before and After Cardiovascular Exercise

If it's your day off from strength training and you're just doing your cardiovascular exercise routine, first warm up for five to ten minutes at a low intensity (50–60 percent of your maximum heart rate) and stretch the muscles you'll be using. Proceed to doing your cardiovascular exercise for at least twenty minutes at an intensity of 50–85 percent of your maximum heart rate. Then cool down for five to ten minutes at a low intensity (50–60 percent of your maximum heart rate). Now, because your muscles are very warm, you should stretch each of the major muscle groups involved in the exercise, using the static stretching techniques I explained previously. For example, if you walked on the treadmill, you should stretch your quadriceps, hamstrings, calves, and lower back. Proper technique for each stretch is absolutely critical for achieving maximum effectiveness in any one specific muscle group. In addition to stretching those muscles used in the exercise, now is also a good time to go through a full-body stretching routine—since blood has circulated throughout your body and warmed up your muscles.

PART III

Buff Workouts for the Essential Wardrobe

WORKOUT 1: BUFF IN A TANK TOP

Tanks should be worn proudly, with arms exposed and bent in a flexed position. Being able to wear a tank top in the summer is like eating a hot dog at a baseball game—it just is! And for some of us, it's become a summertime obsession.

Working the muscle groups of the shoulders, biceps, and triceps is crucial for a sexy tank-top appearance. Training the specific muscle groups that are exposed in the tank top is also crucial to improving your posture. Shoulders that are strong and pulled back, not hunched and rounded, will help you reach your tank-top goal. The following five exercises make a great workout. Remember to complete the number of sets and repetitions appropriate and safe for your level of fitness (1–2 sets for beginners, 3 or more if you are advanced, 8–12 reps each).

OVERHEAD PRESS ON A FITNESS BALL

(Targets deltoids, lower back, and abdominals.)

Sit on a ball, your feet flat on the floor. Maintain a flat back by keeping your abdominals tight. Hold two dumbbells, palms facing out. Elbows should be parallel to your shoulders. Look straight ahead, keeping your head steady. Extend your arms and lift the dumbbells over your head. The dumbbells should nearly touch each other at the extension. Pause, then lower the weights to the starting position. Make sure not to lock your elbows and not to arch your back.

Beginners: 1–2 sets of 10–12 reps
Intermediate/Advanced: 3 sets of 8–12 reps

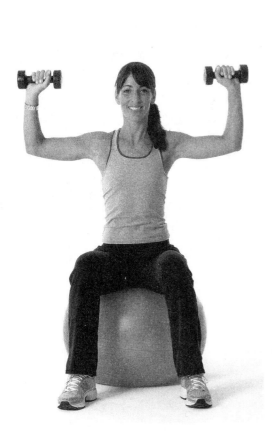
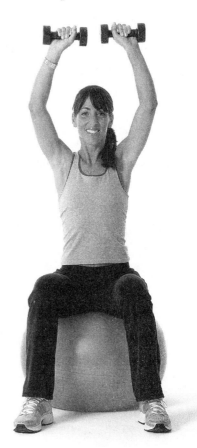

SIDE PLANK SHOULDER RAISE

(Targets deltoids, upper and middle back, legs, and abdominals.)
Place your right hand on the floor, underneath your right shoulder, then
extend both of your legs sideways, placing your right foot behind your
left. Pull in your abdominals so your body forms a straight line from
your head to your heels. Hold a dumbbell in your left hand, arm extended along your hip. Keeping your head and neck in alignment with
your spine, lift your left arm up to shoulder height. Lower slowly to your
starting position. Complete your reps, then switch sides and repeat.

> Beginners: 1–2 sets of 10–12 reps
> Intermediate/Advanced: 3 sets of 8–12 reps

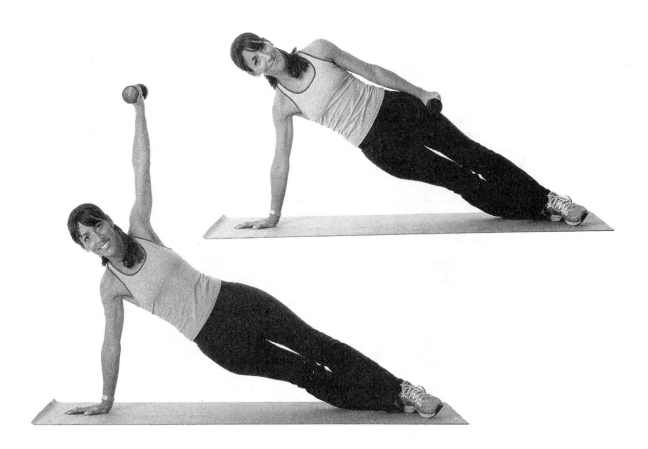

BICEP CURLS ON ONE FOOT

(Targets middle of biceps; core-strengthening move.)
Standing, place your feet shoulder-width apart and hold a dumbbell
in each hand, palms facing in. Lift your right foot off the ground so
your leg is bent at a ninety-degree angle. While balancing on your left
leg, perform a bicep curl; at the top of the movement, your palms
should be facing up. Make sure to keep your elbows locked to your
sides. Slowly lower to your starting position, maintaining your balance
on your left leg. Complete your reps, then switch legs and repeat.

   Beginners: 1–2 sets of 10–12 reps
   Intermediate/Advanced: 3 sets of 8–12 reps

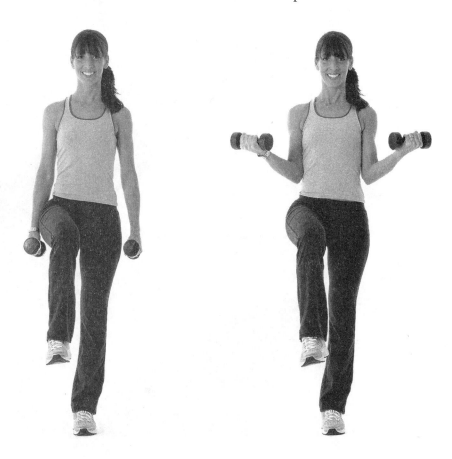

TWO-WAY SHOULDER RAISE

(Targets front and middle deltoids.)

Stand with your feet shoulder-width apart. Make sure not to lock out your knees. Holding a set of dumbbells, arms to your sides and palms facing in, lift your arms up and out to shoulder height. Lower, then lift your arms forward and up to shoulder height, turning your palms up, elbows slightly bent. Lower, turn your palms in, and repeat the combination move.

Beginners: 1–2 sets of 10–12 reps
Intermediate/Advanced: 3 sets of 8–12 reps

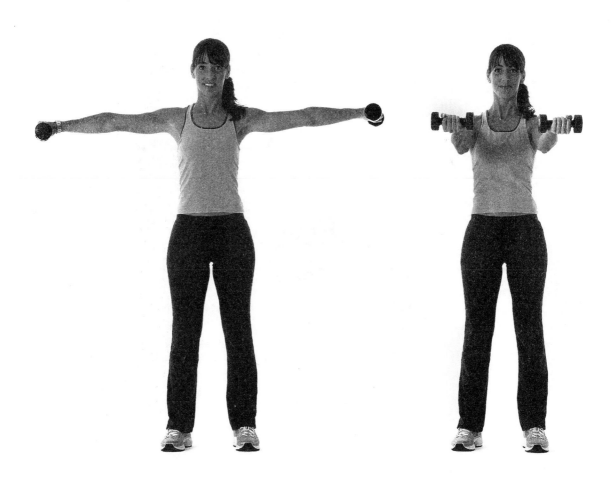

TRICEP DIP WITH A KICK

(Targets triceps, shoulders, glutes, and abdominals.)

Sit on the floor, bend your knees, and keep your feet flat on the floor. Place your hands on the floor with your fingers pointing toward your butt and your wrists aligned with your shoulders. Lift your chest by pressing your feet into the floor. Your hips should be in a low bridge. Straighten your right leg so it's parallel to the floor, foot flexed. Bend your elbows into a dip and lower your hips as you lift your right leg to a forty-five-degree angle to the floor. Straighten your arms, lower your right leg, and raise your hips so you're back in the starting position. Repeat for half your reps, then switch legs.

Beginners: 1–2 sets of 10–12 reps
Intermediate/Advanced: 3 sets of 8–12 reps

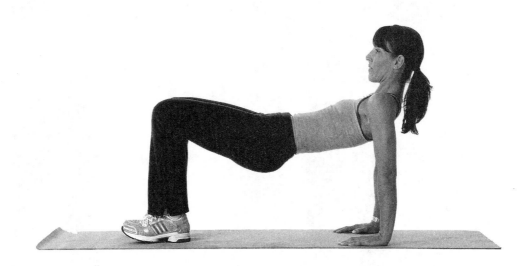

SPORT-SPECIFIC EXERCISES

Yes, there are such things. Sport-specific workouts train the body parts that are crucial for a particular sport. If you want to look great in a formfitting sleeveless shirt and enhance your game of tennis, the tank-top workout plays a dual role. Other sports for which this workout would be helpful are swimming, racquetball, boxing, and gymnastics.

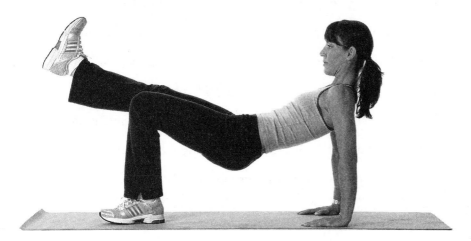

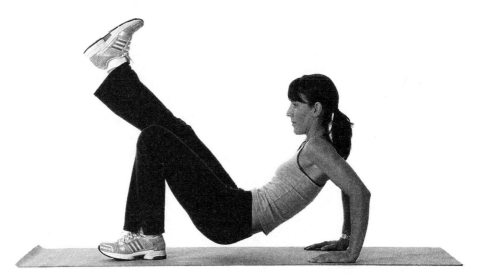

Your butt (or gluteus maximus) is one of the largest muscle groups in your body. (For some of us, *the* largest!) What's known as your glutes covers your entire butt, and its main job is to extend your legs from your hips. Your gluteus medius and minimus are the muscles on the outside of your hip. Women have an especially hard time (except Angelina Jolie) maintaining a fit lower body after giving birth. Getting a buff butt requires you to do some exercises that use all your leg muscles. Try these five exercises for the perfect happy ending!

BUFF WALKS

(Targets butt and legs.)

Standing, hold a light pair of dumbbells at your sides, palms facing in. Take a large step forward with your right foot. As you step forward, your left knee should bend toward the ground, while your right knee stays over your right toe. Return to your starting position and step forward with your left foot.

Walk ten steps forward and ten steps back for 1 set. Repeat for 3 sets.

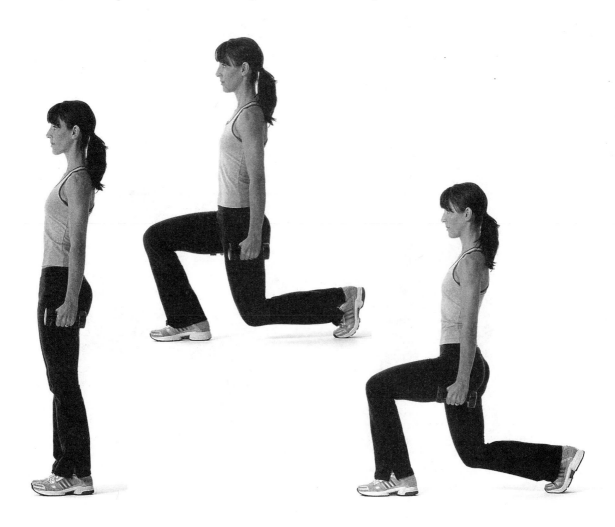

PULSING SQUAT

(Targets butt and quads.)

Stand with your legs two to three times shoulder-width apart. Keep your toes pointed out at a forty-five-degree angle. Sit back and down as if you're sitting in a chair. Slowly lower your butt down about two inches, then return to your starting position. Keep pulsing up and down for 25 repetitions. Then hold the starting squat position for 25 seconds.

Repeat this sequence 10 times.

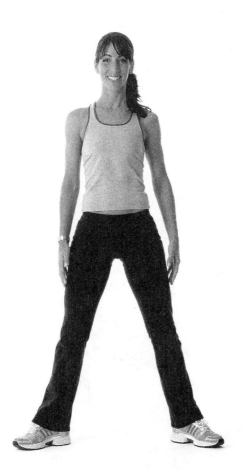
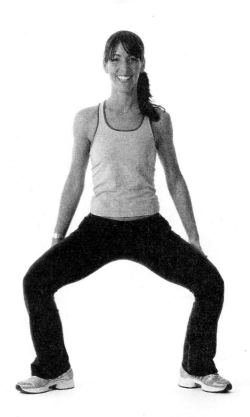

BRIDGE ADDUCTOR

(Targets butt and abs.)

Lie on your back with your knees bent and your feet flat on the floor. Press your hips up into a bridge, creating a straight line from shoulder to knees and keeping your back flat. Extend your right leg and bring it out to the side while keeping your hips up. Aim for 3 sets of 10 reps, then switch legs.

SUPER GLUTES

(Targets butt and abs.)

Place a ball under your pelvis. Place your hands flat on the floor, shoulder-width apart. Tighten your butt muscles (glutes). Raise both of your feet upward, tighten your abs, and hold for two seconds.

Lower and repeat for 3 sets of 12 reps.

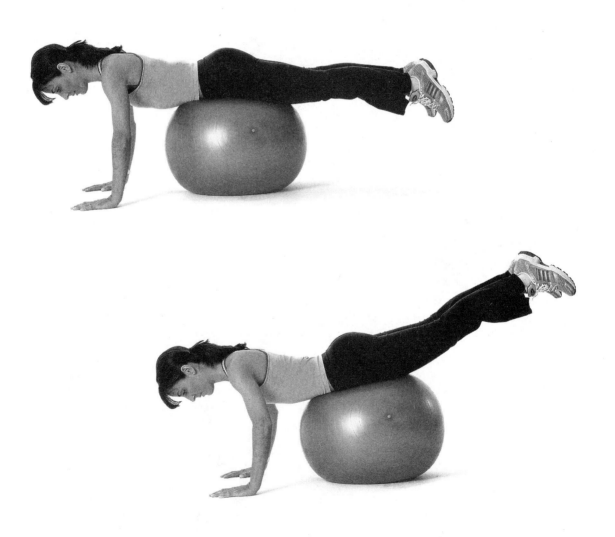

BUTT LIFTS ON A BALL

(Targets butt and core.)

Place a fitness ball under your shins. Walk your hands forward so you are in a push-up position. Your hands should be shoulder-width apart. Keep your back straight and your abdominals pulled in. Keeping your right leg straight and heel flexed, raise your right leg off the ball.

Pulse up and down for 15 reps, and then repeat with the opposite leg. Do 3 sets of 15 reps.

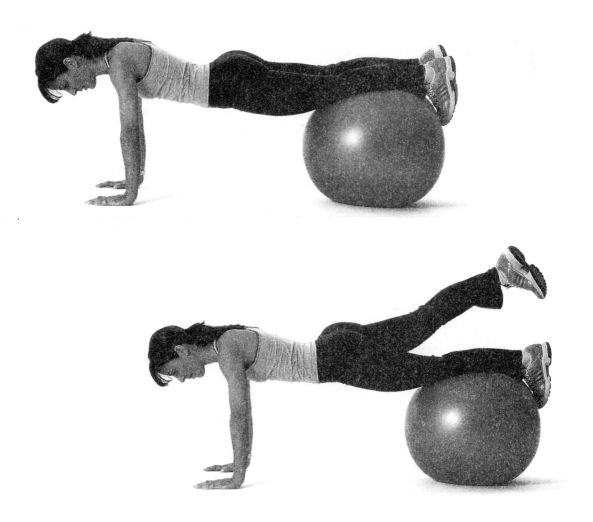

Swimsuit season is right around the corner. Are you ready? Well, if there's one thing women want, it's a tight and toned tummy to show off baring and daring swimsuits. Some say that people are more active in the summer. That may be true, but the menu can also be more appealing during those hot summer months. You've no doubt been to the family barbecues, the countless weddings, and all those other summer events where you crave the less-than-healthy options!

The five abdominal whittlers I outline in this section focus on increasing core strength to give you a better midsection. *Core strength* refers to the muscle groups that stabilize and support your torso while you perform other everyday movements. If these muscle groups didn't exist, you would just fall over.

Doing five hundred crunches is not the way to get a better midsection. Strengthening the surrounding areas is. Building good core and ab strength is the key to a tight tummy. Plus, it helps you work out the rest of your body more effectively. Many folks make the mistake of thinking it's okay to work out their abs every day. The abdominals are muscles, and like all other muscle groups they need time to heal and repair after being worked. Work your abs regularly, but try not to do the same exercise for them daily.

Before we start, let me give you a brief tutorial on the infamous abdominal muscles:

- The obliques run diagonally across your middle. You actually have a pair of muscles on each side. These external and internal muscle groups rotate your torso. They also allow you to flex your torso to the side.

- Typically referred to as the six-pack or washboard, the rectus abdominus is the muscle that all the fuss is about. It's the large muscle that runs from your sternum to your pelvis. Assuming that it's not hidden by fat, the rectus defines most of the front of your midsection.

- The transverse abdominus—the deepest of all the abdominal muscles—is a thin strip that runs horizontally across your abdomen. It's located underneath both the rectus and the obliques, and it acts as a corset to support your entire midsection. It helps keep your organs in place, helps force out your breath, and stabilizes your spine.

TRADE-OFFS

(Targets most of your midsection.)

Lie on the ground and place a fitness ball between your feet. Extend your legs toward the ceiling, squeezing the ball into position with the insides of your feet. Place your arms behind your head. Slowly crunch up, reaching for the ball with your hands. Grab the ball with your hands and slowly bring it down behind your head, keeping your shoulder blades off the ground. Just before the ball touches the ground, contract your abdominals and reach back up with the ball, placing it between your feet. Slowly lower your arms and body back down, again keeping your shoulder blades off the ground. Repeat this move to complete the set (8–12 reps).

Do 1–2 sets if you are a beginner, 3 or more if you are advanced.

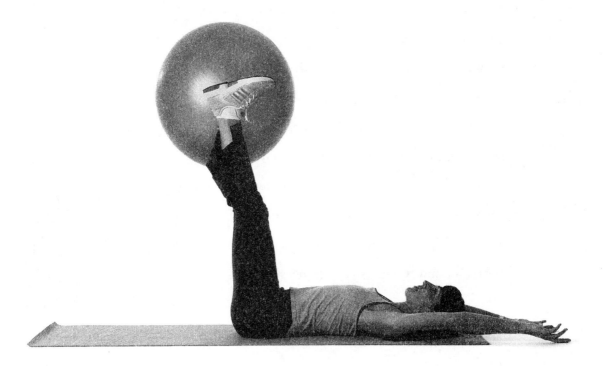

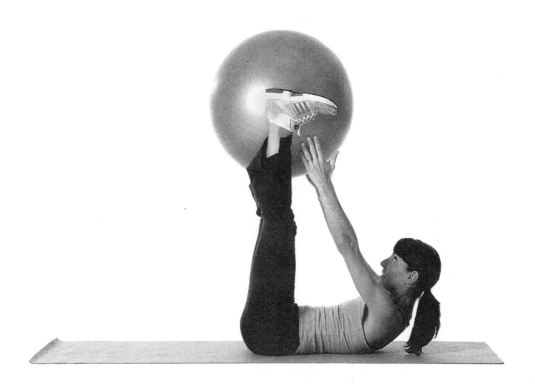

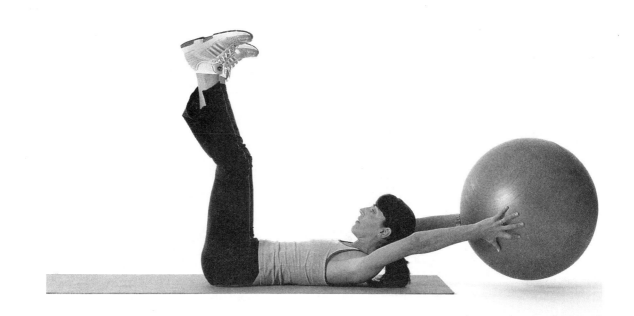

RIGHT ARM/LEFT LEG CRUNCH

(Targets upper abdominals and shoulders.)

Lie on the floor with your legs extended, feet slightly apart. Place a light dumbbell in each hand and raise your arms over your head, resting on the floor. Slowly crunch up, simultaneously raising your right arm and your left leg until they meet over your torso. Once the dumbbell meets your left shin, slowly lower to your starting position. Repeat this move, crunching up so your left arm meets your right shin (8–12 reps).

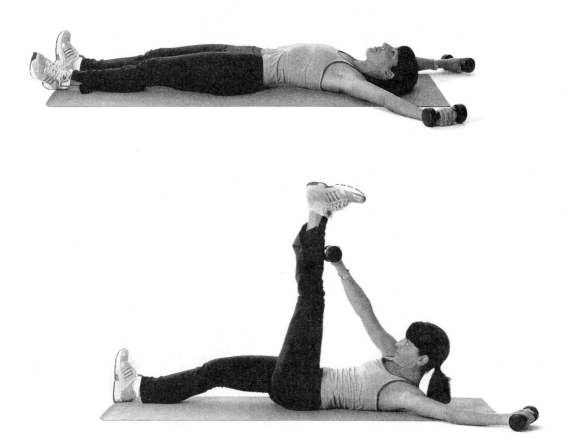

FITNESS BALL AB PULL/PUSH-UP COMBINATION MOVE

(Targets abdominals and upper body.)

Get into a push-up position and place your toes on the ball, keeping it behind you. With your abdominals tight, pull the ball in toward your chest with your feet, then roll it back out. Slowly bend your elbows and lower your body to perform a push-up. Keep your abdominals contracted throughout. Repeat this combo move, starting with the ab pull (8–12 reps).

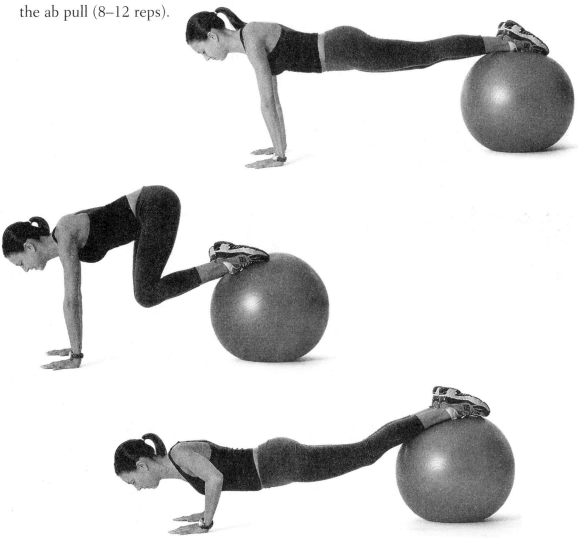

BALL PIKE

(Targets abdominals and spine extensors.)

Kneel behind a fitness ball, then put your body over the ball and walk your hands forward to a plank position. Your arms should be in line with your shoulders, shins on the ball, legs straight, and feet together. Tighten your body, especially the core muscle groups. Contract your abdominals, flex at your hips, and draw the ball under your torso, pulling with your legs and feet. Keep your legs as straight as possible. Focus on bringing your hips toward your ribs so as not to place too much weight on your shoulders. Slowly return to your starting position. Do 8–12 reps.

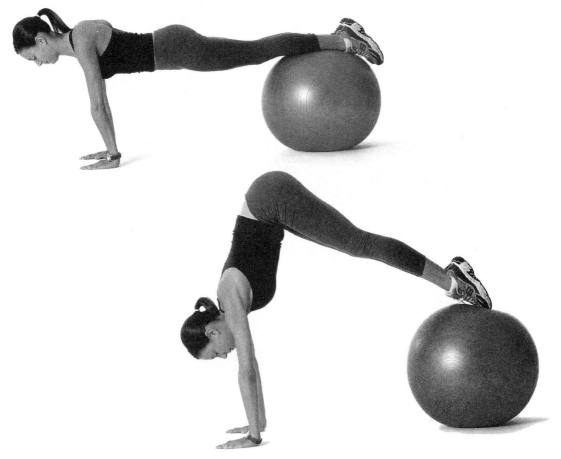

FITNESS BALL WEIGHTED TWIST

(Targets upper and lower abdominals and obliques.)
Sit on a fitness ball; place your feet flat on the floor. Roll forward until the ball is situated on your lower/middle back. Hold a light dumbbell vertically with your arms straight out in front of you. Lean back slowly, being careful not to go too far. Contract your abdominals. Twist your torso up as far as you can to one side and then to the other to complete a rep. Do 8–12 times.

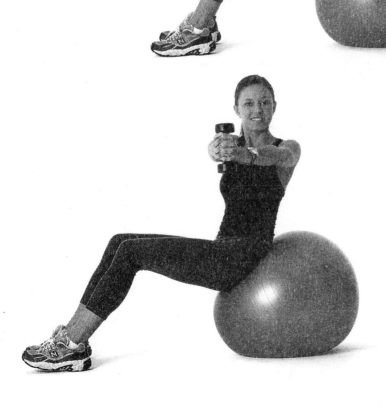

The exercises described on the following pages focus on all the areas of the body that are exposed or emphasized in a little black dress.

X ROTATION

(Targets obliques, quads, butt, and outer thighs.)

Stand with your feet shoulder-width apart, knees slightly bent. Hold a five-pound dumbbell in each hand. Keeping your shoulders, head, and arms facing forward, jump both legs at a forty-five-degree angle to the right side, staying in a semi-squat position. Then jump your feet 180 degrees to the left side, keeping your body and arms facing forward.

Repeat for thirty seconds, then rest and repeat for 3 sets.

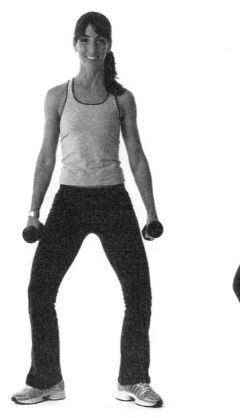
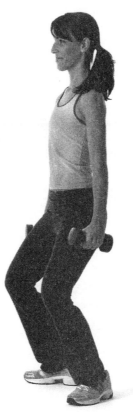
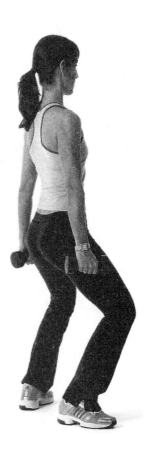

PUSH-UP WITH MOUNTAIN CLIMBER

(Targets chest, shoulders, triceps, and legs.)

Get into a full push-up position, forming a straight line from your head to your heels. (To modify, place your knees on the floor.) Bending your elbows, lower your chest toward the floor. Push up and repeat for 10 push-ups. Keeping your palms on the floor under your shoulders, and your hips low, jump your left knee in toward your chest. Continue to alternate legs for ten seconds.

Repeat the push-up/mountain climber combo for 3 sets.

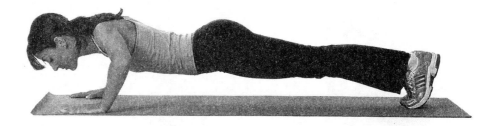

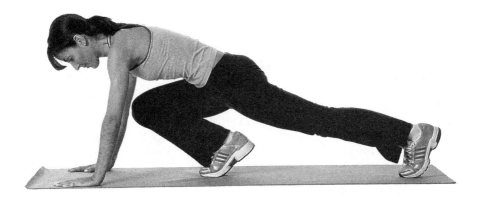

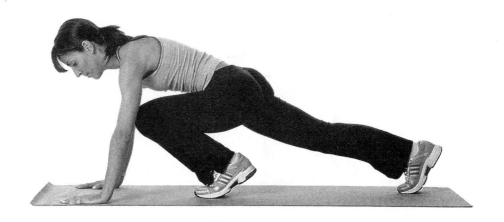

WOOD CHOPPER

(Targets obliques, shoulders, and legs.)

Stand with your feet about shoulder-width apart and grasp a light dumbbell in both hands, holding it outside and above your right shoulder. Flex your knees slightly and pull in your abs. Keeping your elbows bent slightly, pull the dumbbell diagonally across your body until it's beside your left hip. Reverse direction, returning to the start.

Repeat for 10 reps, and then switch sides. Do 3 sets of 10 reps.

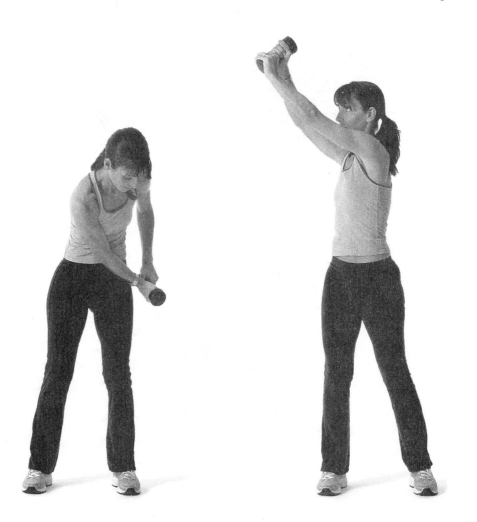

FITNESS BALL PREACHER CURL

(Targets biceps and shoulders.)

Place a pair of dumbbells on the floor in front of a fitness ball. Kneel directly behind the ball and drape your arms over it to grab the dumbbells in an underhand grip. Let your weight move back toward your heels as you brace your triceps on the ball. Keep your back straight as you curl the weights up until your forearms are just short of perpendicular to the floor. Slowly lower, making sure not to use momentum to lower the weights.

Repeat for 3 sets of 12 reps.

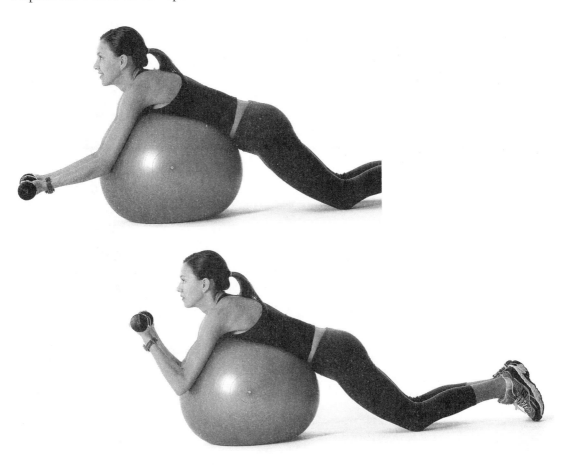

DUMBBELL SPLIT SQUAT WITH A BICEP CURL

(Targets leg muscles, especially quadriceps, as well as biceps.)
Hold two dumbbells in your hands, palms facing in. Stand with both
feet together, then take a giant step forward with your right leg. Your
left heel will lift off the floor. Drop your body weight downward by
bending your right knee and lowering your left knee toward the floor.
As you press back up to a standing split (straightening your legs, but
keeping them wide apart), perform a bicep curl. Make sure to keep
your elbows pressed into your sides. Repeat the drop, completing all
sets on one side, then switch legs.

Do 3 sets of 10 reps.

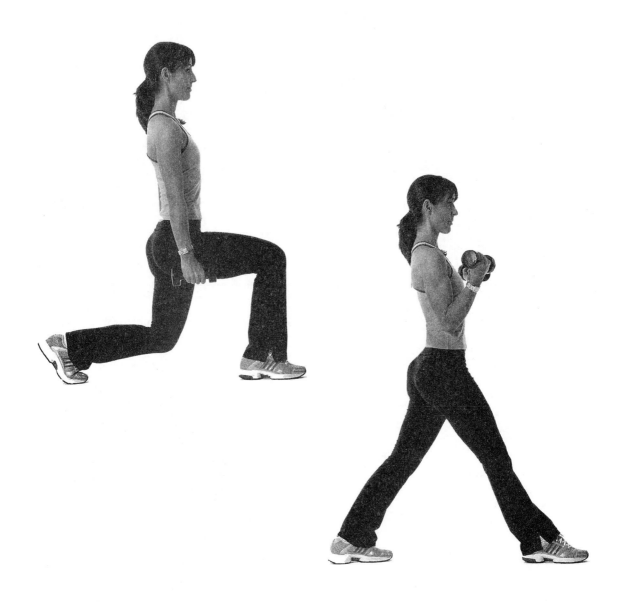

It's almost impossible to flip open a magazine or newspaper these days without seeing a model posed glamorously—if precariously—atop four- or five-inch heels. Yes, it seems that the stiletto heel, along with the platform shoe, has made a comeback in the world of high fashion. A common complaint of my female clients is the leg pain they experience after a day or night of high heels. Strengthening the major muscle groups of the legs will help to alleviate this problem to some degree.

The following exercises will strengthen your calf and leg muscles, as well as help to strengthen your back and abs—two other areas crucial for heel wearers.

FORTY-FIVE-DEGREE TRAVELING LUNGE

(Targets adductors, glutes, and quadriceps.)
Stand with your feet hip-width apart holding two dumbbells at your sides. Lunge forward with your right foot, stepping out at a forty-five-degree angle. Your right thigh should end up parallel to the floor, with your right knee over your toes. Step forward with your left foot, ending up in your starting position. You should have traveled forward at an angle. Repeat the same motion, now stepping forward with your left foot. Keep alternating until you complete a set (8–12 reps). Do 1–2 sets, or 3 or more, depending on your fitness level.

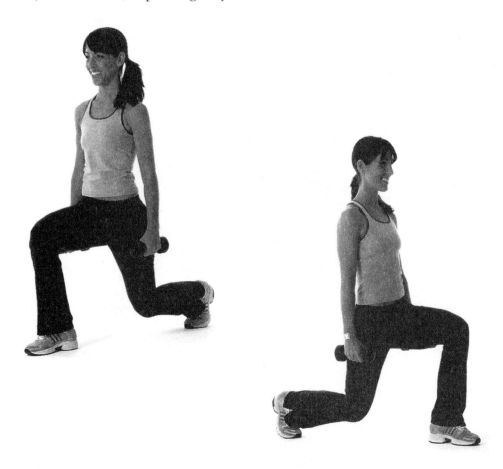

CALF RAISES WITH A BALL

(Targets gastrocnemius, or calf.)
Place a fitness ball against a wall and place your chest on the ball. Keeping your feet together, hold a dumbbell in each hand, palms facing in. Slowly rise up onto your tiptoes (as high as you can go), keeping your ankles stable. Pause for three seconds, then lower to your starting position. Do 1–3 sets, 8–12 reps.

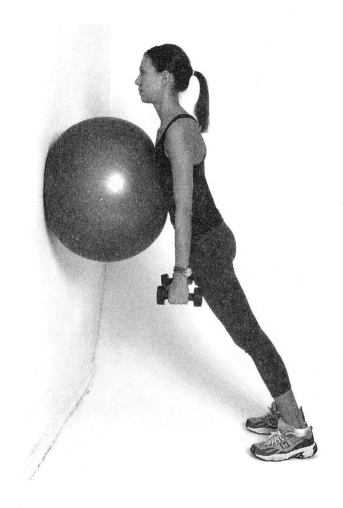

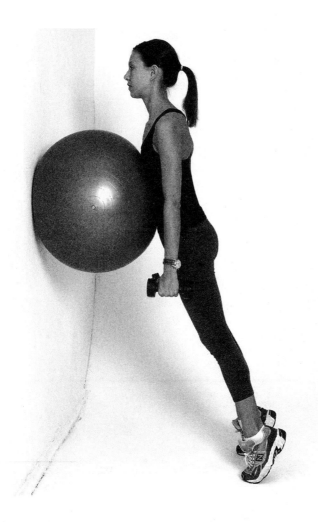

DON'T FORGET YOUR LOWER BACK!

What do lower-back pain, midback pain, upper-back pain, and headaches all have in common? They can all be caused by wearing high heels on a regular basis. Make sure to include the following two back exercises in your stiletto heel workout.

BIRD DOG

(Targets lower-, mid-, and upper-back muscles.)

Start on all fours, with your knees and toes on the floor and your palms facedown in front of you. Pull in your abs, then straighten one arm and the opposite leg, extending both parallel to the floor while keeping your abs tight and your hips in line with your abs. Hold for three seconds. Lower, then repeat on the opposite side, which completes 1 set.

Repeat for 3 sets of 12 reps.

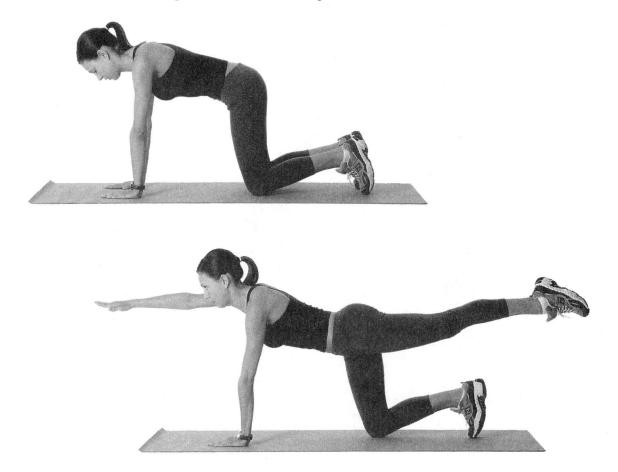

PALM ROTATION ROW

(Targets muscles in middle and lower back, as well as rear deltoids.)

Grasp a dumbbell in each hand with an overhand grip and straighten your arms. Bend over and bend your knees, keeping your lower back straight and your chest out. Lift the dumbbells to each side of your torso, twisting your palms as you lift so your palms face forward at the top. Your elbows should be moving straight toward the ceiling as they bend. At the top of the exercise, reverse the movement, twisting your hands into an overhand grip.

Repeat for 3 sets of 12 reps.

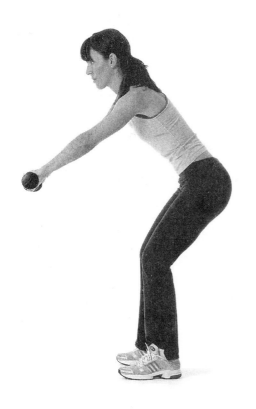
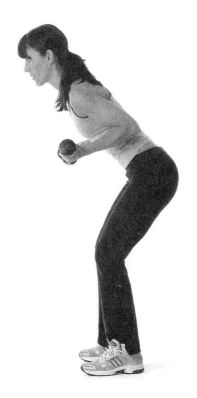

DON'T FORGET YOUR ABS, EITHER!

Yes, strong abs are just as important as strong calves when wearing high heels. Lower-back pain that is associated with wearing heels usually means that your ab strength and lower-back strength are out of balance. This ab exercise will help.

HIP THRUST

(Targets lower abdominals.)

Lie faceup on the ground with your arms spread slightly, palms down to provide balance. Lift your legs to nearly perpendicular to the ground. Raise your hips and butt straight up off the ground by using your abs. Try to touch the ceiling with the soles of your feet, then lower your hips to the starting position.

Repeat for 3 sets of 15 reps.

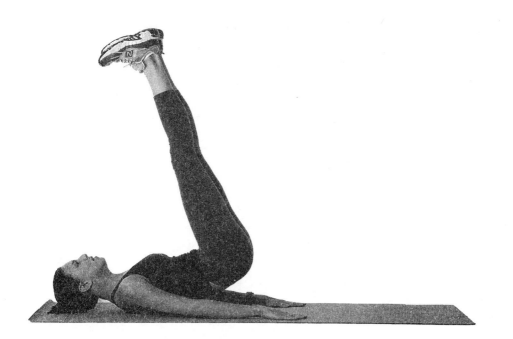

We've all heard of the dreaded "thankels" disease. You know, when the out-of-shape thigh runs right into the ankle? There's basically no muscle definition at all, just one long, flabby thing hanging from the base of your hip. Well, thankels no more! With all the large muscle groups found in the lower body, you can work this area more effectively and efficiently than other areas.

THE SIDE LUNGE

(Targets quadriceps and inner-thigh, or adductor, muscles.)
Hold two dumbbells on the sides of your body, palms facing in. Your
feet are together. Step two feet out to your right side, keeping your
toes pointed forward as your knees bend into a side-squat position.
Keep your butt low, aiming to keep your knees over your toes. Push
yourself up back to the start and finish your reps before switching to
your left leg.

Do 2 sets of 10 reps.

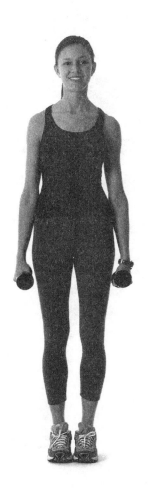
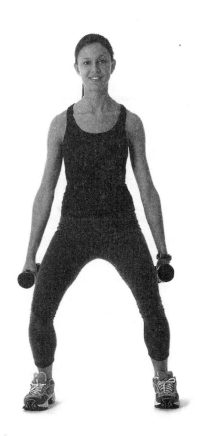

SINGLE-LEG SQUATS

(Targets quadriceps and butt.)
Stand with a fitness ball between your lower back and the wall, feet shoulder-width apart. Maintaining a neutral spine, flex your right leg at the hip and knee to lift your foot from the floor. Squat on your left leg (no lower than ninety degrees), hold for three seconds, and return to the standing position.

Repeat for a set of 12 and then switch legs. Do 3 sets of 12 reps.

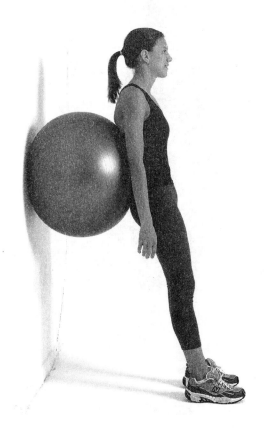

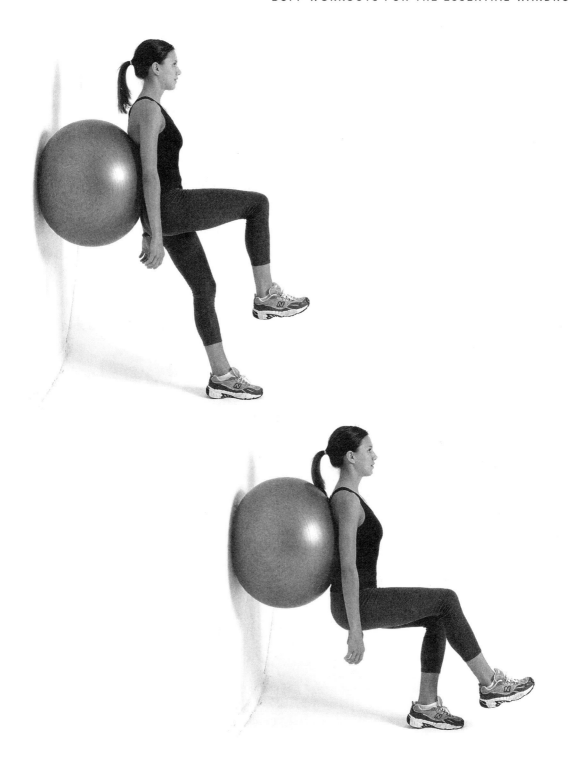

SUMO SQUAT

(Targets quadriceps, butt, and inner thighs.)

Take a wide stance—twice the width of your shoulders—and point your toes slightly out. Pick up a heavier dumbbell with both hands and extend your arms down so the dumbbell is pointing toward the floor between your legs. Pull your shoulder blades back and keep your back straight. Bend your knees and lower your body until your thighs are parallel to the floor. Try to keep your knees over your toes as you lower your body.

Do 3 sets of 12 reps.

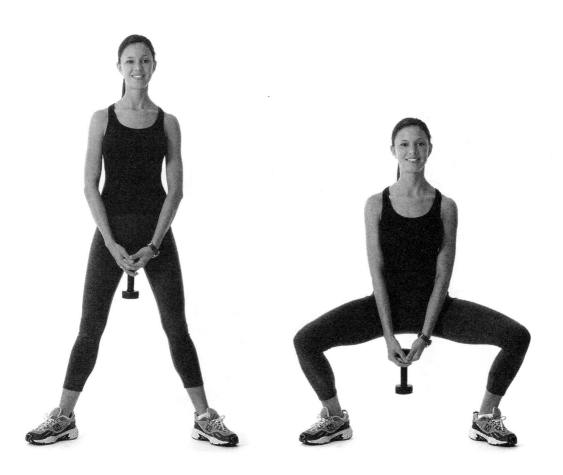

Six Weeks to a Buffer Body!

This routine not only will get your heart rate up, but will also give you a great muscular workout. The following series of exercises hits most of the major muscle groups, so if you want an overall workout, this is for you! Do this combination four times per week, and after six weeks you will be the owner of a firmer, buffer body.

Even though this workout includes a cardio component, for a bonus add twenty to thirty minutes of your favorite cardiovascular activity. See pages 61–64 for suggestions.

JUMP POWER LUNGE

(Targets quadriceps, butt, hamstrings, and lower back.)
Stand in a staggered lunge, left foot forward, right leg behind you.
Jump straight up and switch legs in midair so you land with your legs
in the opposite positions.

Do 15–25 jumps.

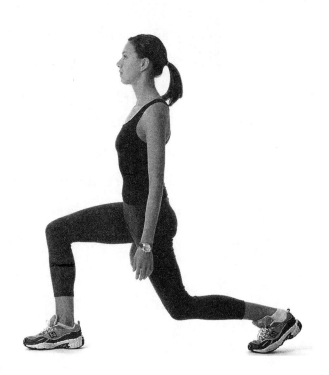

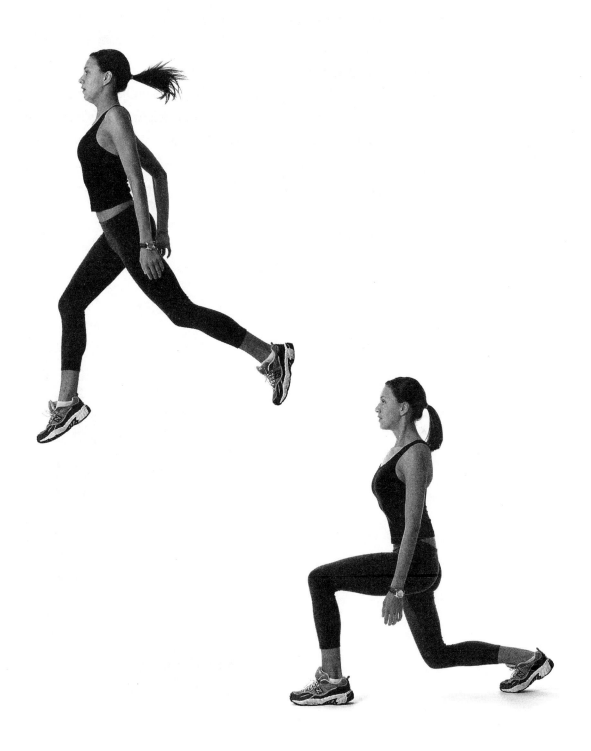

STEP-UPS WITH AN OVERHEAD PRESS

(Targets quadriceps, butt, and shoulders.)

Stand in front of a step and hold a dumbbell in each hand, with elbows bent at ninety degrees, hands up at shoulder height, palms facing out. Step up onto the step with your right foot; at the same time, lift the weights above your head in an overhead press motion. Slowly lower your body and your arms back down to your starting position and repeat with the same leg.

Work each leg for 3 sets of 12 reps.

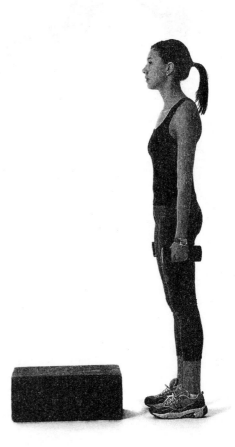

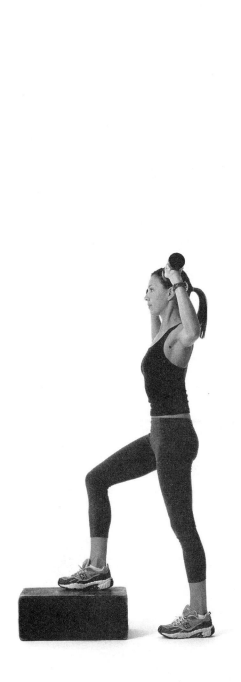
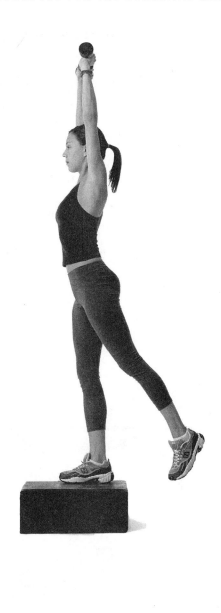

DUMBBELL PUSH-UP AND ROW

(Targets chest, triceps, shoulders, upper back, and abs.)
Place two dumbbells about shoulder-width apart on the floor. From a push-up position, your feet should be shoulder-width apart. Align the weights directly below your shoulders and grip them securely. Lower your body to do a push-up; your back should remain straight, and your abdominals in. Beginners may need to start on their knees. Press back up until your elbows are fully extended. Shift your body weight to your right arm and row the left dumbbell up to your left side. Lower the dumbbell and repeat on the other side.

Repeat for 2 sets of 10 reps.

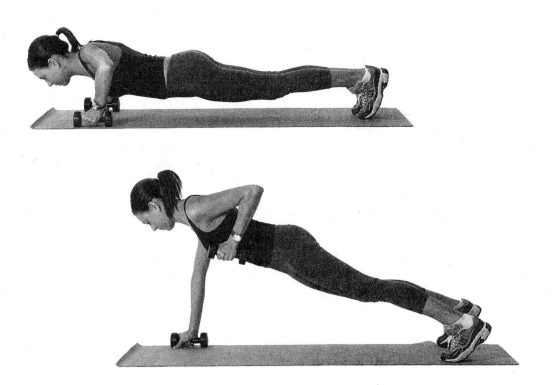

ONE-LEG TOUCH AND BICEP CURL

(Targets **quadriceps, hamstrings, butt, shoulders, and biceps**.)
Stand with your feet hip-width apart, holding a dumbbell in each
hand. Raise your left foot behind your body, balancing on your right
leg. Squat down, touching the weights onto the floor on either side of
your right foot. Stand, lifting your left knee in front of your body while
curling the weights toward your chest. Keep your elbows tucked in to
the sides of your body.

Do 10 repetitions, then switch legs. Complete 3 sets of 10 reps.

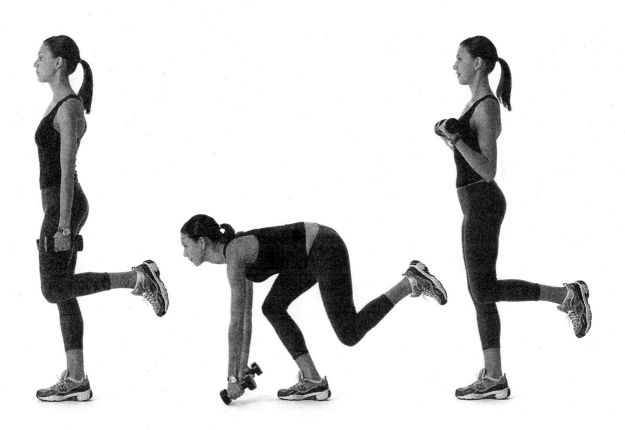

SQUAT THRUST

(Targets butt, quadriceps, hamstrings, calves, lower back, and abs.)

From a full push-up position, jump your feet forward, landing outside your hands. Jump up to a standing position, reaching your hands toward the ceiling. Squat down, placing your hands on the floor shoulder-width apart. Now jump your legs back to a full push-up position.

Repeat for 3 sets of 12.

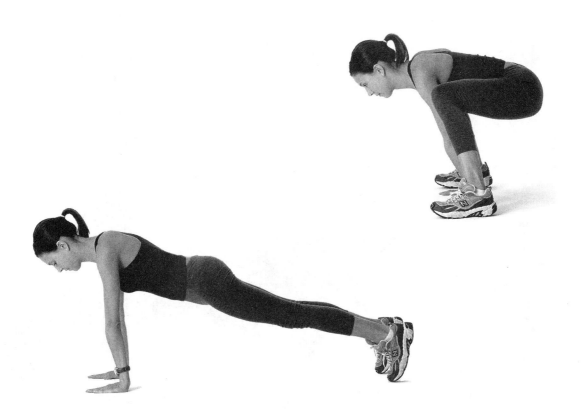

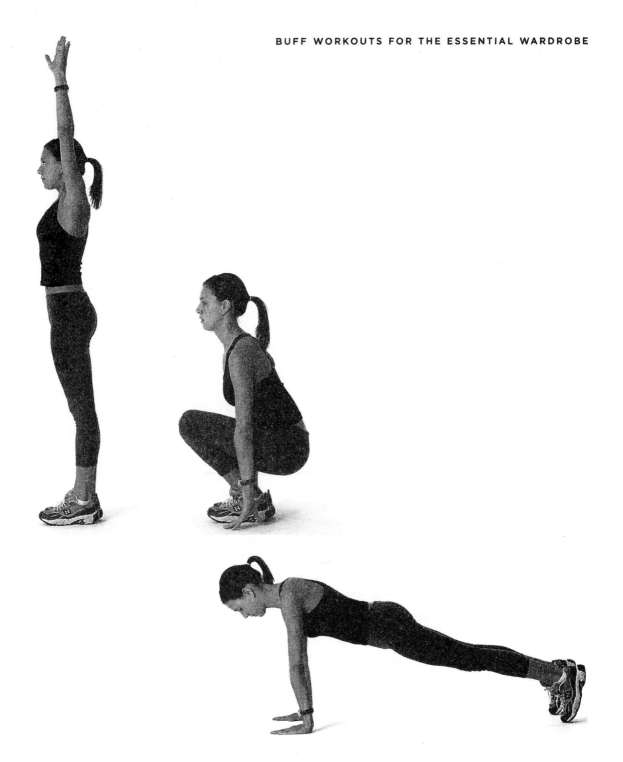

Congratulations! You are now fit, fashionable, and *Buff*!

ACKNOWLEDGMENTS

I am deeply grateful to a number of people for their help in publishing this book:

At Villard/Random House, thank you to my exceptional editor, Danielle Durkin, for her expertise, feedback and support—I so appreciate everything you do.

Many thanks to Bruce Tracy, Kate Blum, Sarina Evans, and Robin Schiff.

A special thanks to Andy McNicol and Jennifer Rudolph Walsh at the William Morris Agency.

I would also like to thank the following people, whose hard work made this book a reality: designer Jack Myers, for his vision and creativity in the interior design; photographer Kelly Campbell, for her keen eye and beautiful work for both cover and interior photography; and models Nicole Boruchin and Erin Bloete.

I'd also like to thank all of the wonderful people at the Inspired Corporation for their efforts to push Buff to another level. Thank you to Jonathan Stathakis, Donald Kasen, Stephanie Hunter, Danielle Kasen, Laura Smith and countless others who have given many hours to support me and the Buff brand.

Also thank you to MagRack, especially Cyndy Cecil and Michelle Adler.

Finally, I would like thank all of the wonderful family and friends who continue to suport me on this journey, especially my friend and lawyer, Karen Shatzkin, all of the wonderful people and members of my department at the Riverdale Country School, Greg and Leigh Anne Brodsky, Lauren Van Kirk, my little cousin Pammie Gryer, Aunt Florence and Uncle Steve Guyer, Bonnie Eldon, Deb Larkin, Suzanne Borda, Anita Cochran, Sandy and Floss Frucher, the Koss-DeFrank family, Eric Lee, Jesus Escobar, Julian Walker, all of my dedicated and fantastic looking clients, and finally, thank you to Kate Frucher for the many years of love and support.

INDEX

bicep exercises (*cont.*)
    split squats with bicep curls,
      102–4
bicycling, 63
bikinis, *see* swimsuits
bird dog exercise, 108
boat-neck styles, 9, 10
body types
    apple-shaped, 6, 7, 8, 12
    and jeans cuts, 15–17
    overview, 5–7
    pear-shaped, 6, 7–8, 11–12, 16
boots
    and boot-cut jeans, 11, 12, 17
    and cropped jeans, 16
    with straight skirts, 12
bottom-heavy, *see* pear-shaped body
    type
bottoms, for pear-shaped body type,
    11–12
    see also jeans; pants; shorts; skirts
bridge adductor exercise, 85
broad shoulders, 10
buff walk exercise, 83
bust and chest exercises
    best bikini styles, 21–24
    neckline considerations, 10
    push-ups, 98–99, 124
butt, *see* gluteous maximus
butt lifts, 87

C
calf exercises
    calf raises, 106–8
    squat thrusts, 126–27
    see also leg exercises
Capris, 16

cardio sessions
    combination of activities, 58
    frequently asked questions,
      56–58
    overview, 57–58
    popular options, 61–64
    and target heart rate, 58–61
    warm-ups, 61
    workout length, 56–57
cargo pants, 11
cargo shorts, 31
clam digger pants, 16
classic-rise jeans, 15
clothes, for working out, 52–53
cowl-neck styles, 9, 10
crew-neck styles, 10
cropped jeans, 15–16
cutoff shorts, 31

D
daily workout logs, 53–54
deltoid exercises
    overhead presses, 76
    palm rotation rows, 109
    side plank shoulder raises, 77
    two-way shoulder raises, 79
double chins, concealing, 9
dresses
    for apple-body type, 12
    basic black, 25–28
    and boots, 12
    empire, 8, 26
    halter, 27
    lace, 27
    long-sleeved, 26
    for pear-shaped body type,
      7–8

About the Author

Fitness expert SUE FLEMING is the creator of the Buff Fitness workout regimen. The program's popularity led to the critically acclaimed reality-TV series *Buff Brides.* She is also the author of *Buff Brides, Buff Moms-to-Be,* and *Buff Moms.* For more on Sue Fleming, including information on her new line of Buff workout DVDs, visit www.fashionablybuff.com.